Core Healing

Dissolving the Dis-eases of Our Times

Joyce Fern Glasser, Ph. D.

Heart of the Golden Triangle Publishers

Published by:

Heart of the Golden Triangle Publishers

Eustis, Florida

Copyright 2007 by Joyce Fern Glasser, Ph.D.

First Edition

ISBN 978-0-615-16597-4

Original cover art work by Diane Romanello; Dartist2@aol.com

Logo design: Inspired by Gold in Art Jewelers; www.goldinart.com

For comments to the author, scheduling interviews, seminars or speaking engagements, contact through www.drjoyceglasser.com

Printed in the United States of America

All rights reserved. Written permission must be secured from the publisher to use or reproduce any part of this book, except for brief reviews or articles.

Dedication

In Loving Memory of My Parents

Sylvia Glasser
Daniel Glasser

With Everlasting Gratitude

Joyce Ann Morris
Pamela Hutul Ross
Madelaine Frishman
Shirley Ellen Anderson

With Humble Admiration

Mahatma Gandhi
The Reverend Martin Luther King Junior
The Dalai Lama

With Special Love

Mary Glasser Paladino
Emily Glasser Susman
Daniel Robert Glasser

CONTENTS

About the Author V
Introduction Vi

PART 1:
CORE HEALING

1. New Hope for Healing 1
2. Our Two Minds: How they Work, Who is in Charge 12
3. How We Become Who We Are (And How Dis-Ease Develops) 22
4. Our 10 Core Fears, Negative Self Concepts and Beliefs 45
5. Core Healing: What It Does 61
6. The Core Healing Process: How It Works 71

PART 2:
Dissolving the Dis-eases of Our Times

7. Depression 92
8. Anxiety 103
9. Stress Management 111
10. Substance Abuse 119
11. Eating Disorders: Obesity, Anorexia, and Bulimia 128
12. Purposelessness 141
13. Unhealthy Attractions 147
14. Anger Resolution 157
15. Physical Problems 167
16. Habit Control 175

ABOUT THE AUTHOR

Joyce Glasser, Ph.D., presents here a process that her client's speak of as "core healing." From her earlier career as an educator, she is the author of *The Elementary School Learning Center for Independent Study*.

She has practiced psychotherapy in Florida since being licensed as a mental health counselor in 1982. Before returning to school at age 39 to get her Ph.D. in Educational and Clinical Psychology at Florida State University, she enjoyed an eighteen-year career as an educator. She holds a M.Ed. in Educational Administration from the National/Lewis University and a B.A. from Lake Forest College. She has taught graduate level extension courses for the National/Lewis University.

Dr. Glasser lectures, leads seminars, has made frequent radio and television appearances, conducts a thriving practice, has developed an adapted Core Healing process for 16-17 year olds, and trains mental health professionals in Core Healing.

She can be contacted through her web site at: www.drjoyceglasser.com

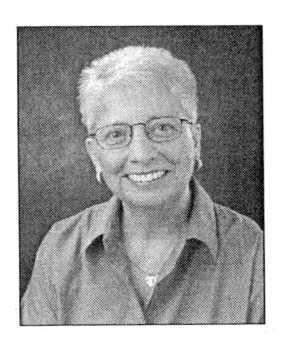

Introduction

I debated about entitling this book Core Healing as there are others out there who refer to what they do similarly. Some use this terminology in physiological context. Words such as homeopathy, deep massage therapy, and acupuncture are embraced in such context. One whose work I read, refers to what she does as Core Belief Psychotherapy, (Brown, 2007).

Core Healing, as described in this book, provides the benefit of doing twenty years of *hypnoanalysis*. These twenty years of hypnoanalytic work in the domain of the subconscious mind, a person's computer center, has provided a wealth of understandings that all these worthy therapies simply cannot provide. It is these understandings that are presented here. It is these understandings that have the potential for changing the DNA (Rossi, 1976), let alone the quality of life for an individual. That is Core Healing.

Core Healing evolved naturally over my career as a therapist, and also through my journey as someone who wrestled with eating and anxiety issues. I discovered its principles and techniques gradually, both as client and as practitioner, and began putting them together in a way that produced extraordinary results for hundreds of my clients over the past twenty years.

I had personally experienced traditional therapy for anxiety when I was an educator. In 1982, I changed careers and became a therapist myself. By 1984, I weighed 200 pounds and felt completely out of control with my eating. Hypnosis was becoming popular at the time so I decided to give it a try.

The hypnotherapist, using the issue of my eating out of control, led me back to a relevant memory while in the hypnotic state. It was a time when I was six years old. Our family lived in Chicago. One afternoon we were sitting around the family room that my father had finished in knotty pine. My Uncle turned to me and as he so often humiliatingly said, "What's the matter with you? Why can't you get rid of that baby fat? You're old enough now."

I was angry. I felt embarrassed and out of control of the situation. Children didn't talk back to adults in those days, so I didn't say anything. Instead, I got on my bike, rode down to the corner drugstore, sat at the soda fountain, and ordered a pineapple ice cream sundae. I turned to something outside myself—in this case, sweets—to take back the control. And I continued to do that well into adulthood. Whenever I felt out of control, I used food to take back control. Of course, that meant that I ate more. The weight packed on. When I felt back in control of my life,

I slimmed down. It was a classic case of yoyo weight gain and loss.

In reaction to my Uncle, I had made a rebellious, negative, reactive decision that afternoon. The decision, not consciously remembered, was:"You can't make me!" "I'll eat whatever I want, whenever I want, and, how ever much I want". Seeing that I chose subconsciously to take control in that way, set the stage to change the unwittingly made decision as well as repair my hostile feelings toward my Uncle. This experience was indeed freeing. I walked out of that therapist's office with a wiser decision that left me in substantially better control of my eating. It felt powerful.

I was awed by what was accomplished so easily and in such a short time. That fact caused me to analyze what had happened. This experience also inspired me to learn about this tool called hypnosis, the key that unlocks the door to access the incredible power, the incredible resource of the subconscious mind.

I realized as I analyzed what had happened to me that the subconscious could not only *retrieve* relevant memories, *it was the place to heal them*. When I relived that memory as an adult under hypnosis and interacted with my Uncle as an equal, I got back both my power and my compassion—and I was no longer out of control. A healing took place that involved forgiveness, recovered self esteem, and most importantly, *choices*. I no longer had to eat out of control. I could now pace myself.

Through the marvelous organization called the Florida Society of Clinical Hypnosis, as well as through the parent organization founded by Erickson, I learned a variety of other effective hypnoanalytic and hypnotherapeutic methods. They were integrated into this process. The result is Core Healing.

In holistic fashion, Core Healing includes five areas for attention and resolution for every client: physical, emotional, spiritual, behavioral, and, in terms of their relationships. This comprehensive approach intends for my clients to enjoy an enhanced capacity to love unconditionally, forgive readily, live responsibly, exude joy, succeed and meet life fearlessly.

Core Healing contains no unique or new components. All are tried and true. What is unique and new is *the way those components are put together in the domain of the subconscious mind*. It is there that thoroughgoing results can most readily be achieved. I have unified resources that my colleagues have been using for decades (such as: Hammond, 1990 and Zarren & Eimer, 2002) around a process that produces deep, universal, and rapid results.

I am grateful to my clients for all that they have taught me, and am especially grateful to those who contributed to this endeavor. Many of the examples in this book are composites of several people's stories, and of course the names and circumstances have been changed to protect their anonymity.

In my mid thirties, I developed a passion to ease pain and suffering in the world. In retrospect, I feel quite confident that it was no accident that I stumbled on this powerful way to bring forward our natural wonderment in such a way as to foster compassion, caring, and unconditional love. So gifted, we can manifest goodness. We can give of our best selves.

And finally, in writing this book, I struggled with who should be the audience - you the public or you my colleagues or both. This book is not of the self help variety that is the typical fare for a lay audience. The Core Healing process requires facilitation by a specially trained professional. It is not a do it yourself project. Therefore, this book is offered to a lay audience from the perspective of education. We are all curious beings and want to know why we are who we are, why do we do what we do, and perhaps most especially, why do we do those things we wished we didn't do, and, what can be done about it.

From a professional perspective, it might have been logical to write about this work in a professional journal first. Regrettably, I do not have the skill required to write in the style required for submission to a professional journal.

Because I was taught during my doctoral studies that it is my professional obligation to pass along what I have learned beyond what is currently known, it is incumbent upon me to write and share such information. It is therefore that I wish to acknowledge that I had help from a professional writer whose skill is writing to a general audience. I am grateful for such help as this book seemed like the next best way to present this work as opposed to the writing skill necessary for presentation in a professional journal. Moreover, at age 69, time feels of the essence.

For you the lay audience, as mentioned earlier, this book intends to educate as well as fascinate you as to how you become who you are, how you function, and, why you behave and feel as you do. For you my colleagues, I sketched the Core Healing process hoping to intrigue you to contact me. Before I cut back my schedule further, my priority will be to teach mental health professionals in the Core Healing process, those already qualified to conduct hypnosis and, who are as excited as I am with such an efficient, effective, comprehensive and relatively brief approach to psychotherapy.

Joyce Glasser, Ph.D.

Chapter 1
NEW HOPE FOR HEALING

This book is about hope. It offers a new way to treat conditions that have seemed mysterious and overwhelming—and to heal those conditions at their source. Core Healing is just that, a deep healing at our very core that lets us thrive physically, emotionally, spiritually, and in our behavior and relationships. Its purpose is to help us enjoy life to the fullest, develop our talents, become the people we are meant to be, attract a bounty of blessings into our lives, and make the contribution we are here to make. Core Healing targets whatever is in the way of doing that.

Depression…anxiety…eating disorders such as obesity…substance abuse…free-floating anger and stress…unhealthy relationships and habits…living with no real sense of purpose…these are some of the dis-eases of our times. We call them dis-eases, of course, because they are the result of "not" being "at ease" within ourselves.

The cost of these dis-eases in dollars and human suffering is incalculable. Worse, they often seem intractable. Each year brings new theories about how to work with them. The best methods researched so far have been a combination of Cognitive Behavioral Therapy and Mindfulness (Begley, 2007). According to Begley, a former science writer for the *Wall Street Journal* but now with *Newsweek* magazine, when dis-eases such as depression are but treated with medication, there is minimal if any resolution. My own experience supports the conclusion that psychotropic medications tend to ease the symptoms as opposed to "curing" the underlying sources of the problems. Be these observations as they may, medication has its place as a crutch and to assist functionality in heretofore unresolvable situations such as Schizophrenia.

Progress in the field of psychology has not been as dramatic as in the field of medical sciences. In my opinion, this slower progress has happened due to the lack of a unified theory of Personality Development. Reconstructing negative aspects of personality is immeasurably more do-able with the working theory I derived from the hypnotic session I experienced. Chapter Three addresses the issue of how we become who we are. Chapter Five discusses the mutability of our personality. That means we are not stuck with what we do not like about ourselves.

So, where do these dis-eases, these conditions. come from? What triggers them? What control do we have over them? Can they be healed without drugs? Can they be healed, once and for all? How can we address their true cause, uproot them at the source, and heal them forever?

The purpose of this book is to address these questions and to offer the hope of Core Healing. I believe not only that life is sacred, but that the quality of our lives is sacred. We don't have to put up with dis-eases that eat away at the quality of our lives. As we heal ourselves, we heal our families, our communities, and thereby the world. We can put a stop to learning and patterning dis-ease behavior from generation to generation, and begin instead leaving an inheritance of hope and healing from a higher plateau of healthy existence.

WHAT IS CORE HEALING?

Core Healing is a process that brings together a variety of widely accepted psychotherapeutic modalities including but not necessarily limited to—aspects of Cognitive Behavioral Therapy, Neuro Linguistic Programming, Inner Child work, trauma therapy, Transactional Analysis, as well as some aspects of Logo Therapy. These therapies are all used in an often unique way in the domain of the subconscious that hypnosis allows. Working in that domain promotes deep, comprehensive, universal, and rapid healing that is not often accomplished through traditional "talk therapy" alone.

By "deep" healing, I mean that issues that have gone unresolved over decades of investigation in traditional therapies are finally put to rest. By "universal," I mean that people often experience more ease, joy, productivity, and well being in *all* areas of their lives—not just those areas they presented as issues and "meant" to heal. By "rapid," I mean that sometimes healing occurs in an instant—but even the most long-standing and difficult issues have the potential of being resolved in four to six sessions. Generally, Core Healing is accomplished in 10.5 to 14 hours. Sometimes the healing unfolds gradually over weeks or months, but it rarely takes the years—and sometimes decades—that more traditional therapies often require.

Core Healing derives much of its power from working with both minds, the conscious and the subconscious which emerges through the use of hypnosis—and from helping these two minds work together in harmony. More often than we realize, the conscious and subconscious minds are at odds with one another. This is what happens when we say we want one thing, but another thing actually happens. We may say we want to exercise more, for instance, but somehow we haven't been to the gym in ages. Our conscious mind knows that exercise makes us look and feel better, and even that it can be fun—but residing in our subconscious can be ideas about ourselves and about life such as "I'm lazy," "I can't take that much time for myself," or "I'm a cream puff; I'll never look or feel that great anyway."

In this kind of battle, the subconscious will win if there are more and/or more onerous negatives against the idea of exercise than for it. It may not be the end of the world if we don't go to the gym, but far more harmful and unproductive ideas are also catalogued in the subconscious—negative self concepts and beliefs that can seriously jeopardize the quality of our lives and even make us ill.

The job of Core Healing is to *identify* the specific negative self concepts and beliefs that generate a dis-ease or condition, *dissolve* them, and *replace* them with their positive opposites—all at the subconscious level through hypnosis. When this occurs, there is harmony between the minds so that we can go forward to thrive, enjoy life more, be more productive, and develop fruitful, nourishing relationships with ourselves, others, and whatever we consider the Divine.

Core Healing is based on twenty years of working with hundreds of patients to produce these kinds of results:

Deb's Depression

Deb had experienced depression for forty years, since the age of four. For ten years, she had sought treatment that included talk therapy and a variety of anti-depression medications. Nothing had worked for her. Under hypnosis, she remembered something that happened when she was four. She had gotten angry and thrown stones at some birds. She accidentally hit and killed one of them. From that day forward, Deb had subconsciously thought of herself as a destroyer of innocent and beautiful creatures, and therefore as a very bad person.

In Core Healing, she was able to see this incident for what it was—a terrible event, but an accident and certainly not something that made her a bad person deserving of eternal punishment. Through a process known as inner child work, these negative self concepts that were imprinted on her subconscious (among them "I deserve to be punished," "I am a bad person," and "I am unlovable") were dissolved. She was led to forgive herself for what happened, and was led through a healing, forgiving conversation with her four year old self and even with the bird. She then replaced those negative self concepts with a sense of herself that was loving, generous, and deserving. All of this was done in hypnosis, so that it took place at the powerful subconscious level.

Deb's depression began to lift immediately, and she now knows how to manage or alleviate it if it recurs. She had no conscious memory of that incident with the bird, and says, "I could have gone on forever, talking about that depression, trying to figure it out, and taking one medication after another. Instead, it's just gone. I have some work to do on some "depressing" (Glasser, William 1976) habits I developed over all those years. But for the first time I can remember, I am free."

Joan's Weight

Joan weighed 295 pounds. She had lost 150 pounds three times using "will power," but the weight always came back. She knew everything there was to know about nutrition, exercise, and weight loss—and wanted desperately, with her conscious mind, to slim down. But she kept gaining. Something was going on beneath the surface, in her subconscious mind, that was overpowering all her good intentions.

In Core Healing, under hypnosis, she discovered exactly what those things were. As a child, she had overheard her mother talking on the phone about a young woman who had been assaulted, telling her friend, "She's so attractive, no wonder they went after her." Joan's subconscious immediately incorporated, "Being unattractive is the only way to stay safe." Over time, she had acquired reinforcing beliefs like "I don't deserve to be happy" and "I'm unattractive anyway; I might as well eat."

No matter what her conscious mind said it wanted, and no matter how much she knew about losing weight, she was fighting a losing battle until she discovered those negative self concepts and beliefs, re-experienced them as an adult, erased them, and replaced them with new, positive beliefs that she was attractive, knew how to be safe without using fat as a fortress, and that she deserved to be loved.

Today Joan weighs 140 pounds. She is active and healthy. She knows she will never regain the weight because she understands and loves herself. She is free and secure, and says, "I can't believe a process that was so painless, and even enriching, could actually change my whole relationship with food and weight—and also let me love myself for the first time I can remember."

HOW IT WORKS

Deb and Joan were living their lives based on negative beliefs about themselves, other people, and the world. Those beliefs had been imprinted on their subconscious minds as a result of traumas early in life, and had gathered around them constellations of related fears and additional and supportive negative beliefs. When their conscious minds wanted something different from what those fears and negative beliefs dictated, they were simply out of luck.

When the conscious mind and the subconscious mind are at odds, the *preponderance* of subconscious self concepts, positive or negative, always wins. (On the other hand, indecisiveness results when the weight of the negatives versus the positives is about equal, or, if there are no relevant self concepts pro or con, or, if there is the self concept of always having to be right. The fear of possible consequence from being wrong can inhibit making a decision.)

I have worked with people who went to extreme lengths to change their habits and behaviors, including gastric bypass surgery to lose weight, but had not dealt with the subconscious negatives that were running the show. Sometimes they lost hundreds of pounds, only to put the weight back on. If those subconscious negatives are not removed and replaced, the body will find a way to act on them—even years later after the gastric bypass surgery!

In Core Healing, we work directly with the subconscious, where those governing factors reside. Hypnosis gives us access to the subconscious, where we identify the specific decisions people have made, delete them, dissolve the negative emotions surrounding them, and lay down positive new beliefs. All of us have hundreds or even thousands of these negative beliefs. Core Healing roots out each one, deletes it, and replaces it with the positive opposite. Positive opposites are a necessary insertion so as not to leave a behavioral void in response to the stimuli that called the negatives into play.

This allows people to exchange fear and anger for love, forgiveness, respect, kindness, and grace. They are guided to stop punishing themselves, and instead go forward as mature adults who can enjoy and contribute to life. They begin to experience peace and serenity, so they can realize their true goals and dreams. My hope is that, as each of us does this for ourselves, and as our lives affect the lives of others, the world becomes a better place.

A client whom I had helped stop smoking, and who works with computers, describes Core Healing this way: "It's like when you want to replace one anti-virus program with another. First, you have to delete the old program. You have to pinpoint exactly where it is in the computer's memory, and then get rid of it so it doesn't interfere with the new program. Only when the old one is gone should you install the new program. Then, when you reboot your computer, it runs the new program—not the old one. If you try to run the new program without deleting the old one, you can get into trouble. So you find, delete, replace, and reboot. Just like I did to become a non smoker."

WHY CORE HEALING IS UNIQUE

I once worked with a psychotherapist on his underlying depression. He had a loving wife and children, but could never really enjoy his blessings. He was quite successful, but was always worried about his practice. Under hypnosis, we identified a childhood trauma he experienced at age six. His father had taken his sister on an outing, and left him behind. It was something he wanted very much to do too. Without his conscious awareness, he had adopted the negative self concept, "I am not enough." He was spending every waking moment trying to prove to himself, his family, and the world that he was bright, able, and *enough*. Since his perception of self was that he could never be enough, as in good enough, his sense of unhappiness lingered.

Under hypnosis, we looked at the incident with his six year old self, and with the person he had been at various other important ages. He talked with his father and told him, adult to adult, in a compassionate fashion, how he had felt. He saw that his not being included had not meant that he was "not good enough," or that his dad didn't love him. He might simply have taken his sister because she was older, or because the father wanted a special afternoon with his daughter, or for a million other reasons that had nothing to do with devaluing him. Next, also under hypnosis, we established some positive alternative beliefs: "I am loveable,"

"I am good enough," "I am a person of integrity and as a man I have value." "My dad is proud of me."

My colleague was amazed at the profound healing he experienced—and even more at the immediacy, comprehensiveness, and the variety of wonderful, tangential outcomes. Since I do not use any techniques that other professionals don't use, and since he was already quite familiar with all the techniques I do use during the Core Healing process, I asked him what the difference was.

"It's the way you put them all together!" he said. "It creates a synergy among the various therapies, and it does so in the subconscious—the part of us that's driving the bus!"

THE PROMISE OF CORE HEALING

We are not stuck with the negative self concepts and beliefs that are behind many of the difficulties we experience in life—physically, emotionally, spiritually, and in our behavior and relationships. Using hypnosis, we can literally redesign aspects of self by unhooking and dissolving negative self perceptions and replacing them with positive beliefs and self concepts.

That process better enables our making satisfying choices. We can choose to live in love, rather than in its adversary fear which can lead to ignoble anger and greed. We can learn from our mistakes, rather than punishing ourselves or blaming others. We can choose forgiveness, and gentleness with self and others, over ugly anger. We can literally alter aspects of ourselves and our personalities that were once thought to be immutable. That way, we are free to be the compassionate beings that sweeten life.

Core Healing works across a broad spectrum of dis-eases because they all happen for the same reason—constellations of relevant negative self concepts and beliefs. When we heal ourselves at the core, it shows up in our relationships, our bodies, our emotions, our spirituality, and our behavior. We heal:

Physically: The most common cause of dis-ease is stress. If we are not carrying fear, anger or pain, and, we feel in constructive control of ourselves, there is no stress in the body.

Emotionally: We can live fearlessly, unleashing passionate purpose and self confidence.

Spiritually: We learn to forgive ourselves, others, and the Divine. We can live responsibly with a sense of gratitude and grace, peace, and an enduring sense of serenity.

Our Behavior: We can release unwanted habits and addictions, regain control of our lives, become responsible for our actions, act with integrity, and access our full potential.

Our Relationships: Desensitizing childhood trauma gives us the ability to have loving adult relationships. At core, under hypnosis, we heal our relationships with our parents and others who may have hurt us, and learn to love ourselves and others unconditionally.

Core Healing renews and reconstructs all five areas because it works at a level that is beneath them all, and senior to them all. The subconscious is at the very core of our being, and most of what ails us is the result of faulty thinking that has developed as negative self concepts and beliefs. We can retrieve ourselves healthfully in all five areas when we heal those negatives.

Core Healing also holds promise on a more global level. Each of us has a core world—our family—that needs to be healed. As we heal ourselves, we raise our own children with less trauma. The quantity of negativity passed from generation to generation could be substantially reduced. As each of us finds peace within our own soul, we are free to love without fear and to become the people we are meant to be—and we can pass on that blessing to everyone we encounter.

Core Healing's Assumptions

Some important assumptions that form the foundation of Core Healing are:
- As you believe, so shall it be.
- Thought precedes everything. My work suggests that there is only one umbrella, overarching category of mental disorder and that is a Thought Disorder. The Diagnostic and Statistical Manual for Mental Disorders IV lists several mental disorders and I would see these as subcategories. It is only from faulty thinking in the form of negative self concepts and beliefs that emotional, physical (psychogenic vs physical handicap as in retardation), behavioral, spiritual and relationship difficulties emanate.
- Your truth, the whole of your truth, and nothing but truth, will set you free.
- Heal the mind, the body follows.
- Much can be accomplished in little time.

- No two people are alike—even identical twins (Harris, 2006).

THE SPIRITUAL COMPONENT

People have asked me if they need to believe in God in order for Core Healing to work. They do not. I believe strongly in a forgiving, benevolent, and divine force at work in the universe. I call it God. Others call it love, the Divine, universal energy, a higher power, or some other name. Core Healing is easier if you believe in such a force or condition—simply because you are more likely to believe that death is followed by something other than a complete void, and that can provide a level of certainty and comfort in times when all other certainty or comfort is absent—but it works even if you do not.

What you must believe in is forgiveness. I used to think that if I forgave someone, it meant that I condoned their actions. There are many behaviors I can't condone—abuse, deliberately hurting someone, cruelty, killing, etc.—but that I can understand and forgive.

Forgiveness simply means letting go of the pain and anger around an event. Without forgiveness, core healing cannot take place.

Some people carry anger with God. It, too, must be dissolved. They must forgive God. If they prayed for God's help with an abuser, for instance, and God did not answer their prayers, then they may be carrying either an anger at God or a sense that they are not worthy of God's help. Their dilemma becomes: Either God is vengeful and unhelpful, or I am so evil that I don't deserve God's help. In either case, they become distant from their spirituality. They must forgive themselves, and also their idea of God, in order to heal. The teachings for our salvation have been made available. Therefore, it is we, not God, who must be responsible for rectification of predicament.

If my clients are comfortable doing so, I ask them to compose a prayer to guide and empower our work together. If they are not comfortable with that, we don't do it—but many people have discovered a latent spirituality, or found that their spirituality took a leap forward, through their experience with Core Healing.

HOW TO USE THIS BOOK

This book is divided into two parts. Part 1 is about Core Healing—the premises and models on which it is based, how negative self concepts and beliefs get imprinted on the subconscious, the top ten core fears that to one degree or another most seem to actualize, and how the process of Core Healing works. Part 2 covers how Core Healing heals specific dis-eases of our times: depression, anxiety, stress, substance abuse, eating disorders (obesity, anorexia, and bulimia), purposelessness, unhealthy attractions, anger, unwanted habits, and physical problems.

You will hear me refer frequently to "conditions," "situations," "issues," and "problems." These types of words are purposely used in an effort to avoid labels such as "Bi-Polar," (the diagnosis du jour) "Schizotypical Personality Disorder," "Anxiety Disordered," or the not so fancy word "addict." To me, "problems" suggest that there is a solution. But authorities labeling people as "Disordered," or "Bi-Polar," or as an "addict" not only entrench such labels as additional negative self concepts and beliefs but these labels gather to them defining concepts that can become whole constellations of relevant, enervating negatives. Such labeling can foster the implementation of the unwanted problem as well as heighten the degree of discomfiting emotion and promote a need for further 'medication'.

People tend to become their labels. Additionally, such labels can even reinforce their negative self perceptions as weak, sick, crazy, a nervous wreck and consequently add to or initiate a sense of hopelessness. Without hope a person at the least feels lost. Without hope there is despair. With despair there can be suicide. Unequivocally, therefore, we must be ever mindful of our words, our labels. *Labels, as applied to the human beings in need of psychotherapy which in a sense means all of us, must be compassionate in tenor, hopeful by design.*

I believe that all the dis-eases we discuss in Part 2 of this book primarily, if not entirely, are manifestations of relevant constellations of negative self concepts and beliefs—but it is important to remember that there is not necessarily a direct correlation between specific negatives and specific dis-eases. In other words, "I deserve to be abandoned" may be common among people who feel depressed, but it will likely manifest among those with an eating disorder, or those who stress their lives so badly with the mismanagement of their personal time that they engage in the release valve of rage, as well as those who smoke. The process of Core Healing is the same, regardless of what condition is being addressed or what negative self concepts are involved.

Is Core Healing for everyone? No. Does Core Healing work for everyone?

No. Be these facts as they are, Core Healing does bring substantial benefits to most people. For Core Healing to work, you must be motivated. You must want to change, be willing to do so, and *believe* that it is possible. The success of Core Healing looks like a bell curve. A very few people on one end are not helped at all. Most people are helped more or less significantly. A few people on the right side of the bell shaped curve have had what might be called miraculous healing and change.

As I train more therapists to use Core Healing, it will become more widely available. My hope is that some of these therapists will take it to even greater heights.

Chapter 2
OUR TWO MINDS:
How They Work, Who Is In Charge

Core Healing owes much of its success to a clear understanding of how the mind works—and to its capacity to access the subconscious, the part of the mind that is in charge. The negative self concepts and beliefs, and all that spawned them, limit us and cause dis-ease to thrive within. Only by working with the subconscious to find, dissolve, and replace the negatives with positives—and by desensitizing the sources of the negatives, can real healing take place.

In this chapter, we will look at the difference between the conscious and subconscious minds, the power of the subconscious, how it can work against our conscious desires, how Core Healing brings our two minds into harmony, and the value of hypnosis in accessing the subconscious to make effective changes. But first there needs to be discussion to differentiate the brain from the mind (s).

The brain is the grey matter housed in our skulls. Its job is sensory reception, interpretation, and response. How well it works depends on genetics, whether or not it is injured, how well it is stimulated and fed, and how it may have become altered by chemicals introduced pharmaceutically, environmentally, or heightened or depressed emotionally, or even altered by an individual's thought patterns.

The mind and the brain can affect one another. The brain affects the mind when, for whatever of the above reasons, it cannot receive, store, access, or interpret data quickly or accurately. The mind can affect the brain when our emotions produce chemicals that alter how the brain functions, or when our thoughts call into play and agitate certain regions of the brain. For instance, an accumulation of negative self concepts can make us feel out of control. Feelings of being out of control, if left to fester and grow, can lead to despair, which leads to the possible suppression of serotonin levels. Serotonin is the brain's "feel good" chemical. Low serotonin levels, in turn, affect how the brain works and exacerbate feelings of depression.

OUR TWO MINDS: CONSCIOUS AND SUBCONSCIOUS

As we have seen, the mind has two parts: the conscious and the subconscious. (The subconscious mind should not be confused with "unconscious," which is what happens when both minds are asleep or "out cold.") The conscious and subconscious minds serve different functions, but are meant to work together as a unit. Only when negative beliefs and self concepts reside in the subconscious, undetected and unaddressed, do the two minds have the opportunity to become dissonant and work against one another.

The conscious mind's job is to evaluate data, and then make judgments and decisions based on those evaluations. It is generally not aware of what is going on with its partner, the subconscious. (In the subconscious mind, a thought, sense or cognition can fly by so quickly that the much slower conscious mind may miss it.) But the subconscious is always aware of what is going on with the conscious mind, which funnels data through all of our senses: sight, smell, touch, sound and taste.

In terms of being aware of who we are, the "everything of us," the conscious mind is just the tip of the iceberg. The subconscious is all the rest, the massive part of the iceberg that is below the surface. If the conscious mind is a peanut of self awareness, the subconscious is a watermelon. Think back to when you were five years old. How aware of the world were you? Your perceptions, knowledge, and understanding were minimal compared to what they are now. We can liken the awareness of a five year old to the conscious mind, and the awareness of an adult to the subconscious. That is why therapies that work only with the conscious mind can produce only a certain level of results.

HOW THE SUBCONSCIOUS WORKS

The subconscious is a vast library or warehouse of information. The data housed accumulates from every aspect of life to which the individual is exposed. From around 'mid-fetushood', through the birthing process and on into life, we gather data about ourselves and our world. Then too, there is the potent infusion of beliefs espoused by our institutions. There are awesome, ever faster and more graphic information sharing tools such as the Internet. We are bombarded with hordes of information and imprinted with powerful images. We are becoming a world community and all that it means for the development of the self concepts and beliefs that shape our personality. While mom and dad remain the key factors of influence upon us, as always, there is also our family especially our siblings and our grandparents and their heritage, as well as other family members. Also of great influence are our communities, our schools, our teachers, our peers, our country, our world. Our places of work have major impact as well. Too many companies encourage uncivilized conduct among staff as well as place huge pressure on the employees and for too little pay. Our houses of worship and their leaders, our sacred texts, all play a major part in our formation as well (Harris, 2006 and Bandura, 1976).

From all walks of life, we accumulate more and more subconsciously housed self concepts and beliefs. Fortunately, our subconscious is an extraordinary computer that houses, organizes and stores vast quantities of data. Instantaneously, we react, respond or create based on a given stimulus. The more sorted out we are with ourselves through such a process as Core Healing, the better able we are not to simply react.

The subconscious does not pause to consider or think about information, as the conscious mind does. It reacts to stimuli in a way that is automated, amoral, and instantaneous. With the speed of light, it orchestrates behavioral, emotional, and/or physiological responses based on the positive or negative self concepts and beliefs contained in its bank of files that are relevant to any given stimulus that requires response.

This bank is enormous, and its files are catalogued brilliantly—unless there is some sort of brain damage. A given stimulus, such as an apple, activates the orchestration of relevant self concepts and beliefs. The generally instantaneous reaction depends on the individual's experience with apples and the relevant self concepts and beliefs gathered around that object. The constellation of beliefs gathered to provide 'appropriate' response depends upon their relevance to the stimulus. A reaction, even a non action, is what results from what the constellation of beliefs dictates. When the stimulus' response is concluded, the components of the constellation are returned each to their own slot in the catalogue. Upon taking in the next stimulus, those self concepts and beliefs that are relevant are ready to be drawn together into a different or similar constellation as they relate to this other stimulus, like a banana. The responses dictated for a person who has a self concept of "I eat everything in sight even if I am full" versus someone who "does not care for fruit" are quite noticeably different.

All positive and negative self concepts and beliefs are stored over the years, and reside in orderly fashion along with the emotional content of each seminal memory. A taste, smell, sight, feel, sound, emotion, or general "sense of things" can stimulate an immediate reaction that is perfectly logical based on the subconscious files, but is not always desirable. The smell of burning wood, for instance, might produce a smile or general feeling of well being if it stimulates the positive self concept of "I am part of a loving family that has enjoyed many a night, sitting around the fire together." But it could trigger fear if, as a child, the person had barely escaped from a burning house and emerged with a subconscious belief that "Burning wood means I'm about to die."

These files, taken as a whole, dictate our behavior in the world—whether or not we remember the seminal events, and whether or not our memories of the events are accurate. The events themselves are not as important as what we *remember* them to be, and what we *make* of them. That is what dictates our reality.

The subconscious does *only* what is dictated by the information it has stored. For instance, the conscious mind may evaluate a student's situation and decide that doing homework is a good idea. But if the student's self concept is that he is "stupid," "lazy," "a failure," and/or "a loser," then it will be nearly impossible for him to do something that is smart, diligent, or that makes him successful or a winner. The subconscious negative self concepts and beliefs will override any fantasy he may have about being an astronaut, an attorney, or a teacher. No homework gets done, no learning takes place, and no dream is actualized.

The subconscious mind even dictates what happens in our bodies. It can create health, or dis-ease. I worked with one woman who had all the symptoms of being pregnant, but was not. She was forty and had her tubes tied after the birth of her third child, something that went against Jewish Orthodox tradition in her particular Chabad (Jewish community). Her subconscious beliefs (that she "should" get pregnant in a let nature take it's course kind of way, and that she deserved to be punished for interfering) caused her body to overcome the effects of the tubal ligation, and the result was her false pregnancy.

After she reconciled the matter at the subconscious level, her sensitive and enlarged breasts and her bloated stomach returned to normal. She lost six pounds in the week following our session with no change in diet. This is one of hundreds of cases that have convinced me: "Change the (subconscious) mind; the body follows."

I believe that the power of the subconscious to affect physical change is virtually unlimited. What resides in the subconscious is not the fault of the individual, so the results of the negatives are not their fault either. It is simply important to acknowledge their existence to rid ourselves of unhealthy effect.

THE INTRA-PSYCHIC BATTLE:
When Conscious and Subconscious Collide

How do the conscious and subconscious minds interact with one another? The conscious mind receives and transmits sensory input, evaluates it, and, makes a decision, if the subconscious hasn't superceded during the slowed time of such process. The subconscious mind then responds and *either allows that conscious decision to proceed, or NOT*—based on its files, our accumulated self concepts and beliefs.

If Greg makes a decision to stop smoking, for instance, a battle may ensue between his conscious and subconscious minds. His conscious mind says, "Quitting is the only logical thing to do. I have high blood pressure and a cough. I know that smoking causes lung cancer. And it's disgusting. I have to go outside at bars and restaurants to smoke, and everyone can smell it on me. Smoking is unhealthy, stupid, and socially unacceptable. I'm going to quit." He tries one smoking cessation program and quits for a week. He tries another program, learns to "white knuckle" life without cigarettes, and stops for seven months. But then he goes back to smoking. Why would he keep doing something that he genuinely believes is bad for him physically, socially, financially, and in terms of his self esteem? What neither Greg nor the people around him—who are all trying to convince him to quit—understand is that his subconscious mind is awash with self concepts and beliefs that simply will not permit him to stop smoking. Among them are:

- "I need to smoke to contain my anger."
- "I am a loner and an outcast."

- "I'll gain much weight and get fat if I stop smoking."
- "I'm going to die young, like my father."
- "Smoking makes me cool and tough."
- "I can't quit because I have no will power."

None of these self concepts and beliefs is necessarily true or logical, and some are obviously false. If you asked Greg if they were all true, he would say, "No! Of course not!" But there they are, and they are running the show, overriding Greg's conscious decision to stop smoking.

Ignorance of how our data processing system works is why it has been so difficult to change behaviors, and why it is usually a waste of time to argue with people about the logic of a better behavior. We assume that people have free will to do what is logically correct, in their own best interest, or in the best interest of society—*but in reality, people can only do what their particular constellations of self concepts and beliefs allow them to do.* They can exercise the power of positive thinking or action only when there are no negatives subconsciously to interfere.

If the conscious mind's decision is not in harmony with the subconscious, an intra-psychic battle ensues—and as we have seen, *the subconscious usually wins*...unless there is a "Mexican stand-off" of negative versus positive self concepts and beliefs that then results in indecisiveness and inaction.

WHOLENESS: RESOLVING THE CONFLICT

Core Healing can resolve conflict that can exist between the conscious and subconscious minds, and bring harmony within ourselves. It does so not only by eliminating negatives in the subconscious, but also because it engages both minds in the process.

The conscious mind of a person identifies the issues that need to be addressed in Core Healing. People choose what they want fixed to the extent the subconscious allows. Based on my experience, I generally suggest additional issues for resolution. I also make sure each client's conscious mind is educated about, and ready for, what we are about to do at the subconscious level. When the conscious mind understands the value of this work, it offers less resistance. I motivate the conscious mind to support the process by convincing it that healing can and will take place—that there is indeed hope. The more hope, the easier that process will be. We also engage the conscious mind to facilitate conversation during hypnosis.

A cornerstone of Core healing is removing the self concept worrier which is aided and abetted by negative thinking such as imagining the worst outcome. Worrying is learned from one or both of our parents or those who raised us. We worry about what they worried about. We simply absorbed their style. It is patterned behavior. Worrying is an enervating, and often immobilizing self concept.

Clients require being educated to the drag down effect of worry and be guided to the alternative style of concern management. One must be action/solution oriented. The conscious mind is also taught to be keenly aware of self talk, and what to do about any negative conversations with self. It too is a major bad habit that is fostered additionally by engaging in self flagellation. Negative thoughts, negative self talk produces negative feelings.

The rest of the Core Healing process takes place in the subconscious. The goal is to align the conscious and subconscious minds so they may work together to heal the problem. When our two minds work together harmoniously, we enjoy serenity and gain the capacity to realize our dreams.

HYPNOSIS: ACCESSING THE SUBCONSCIOUS

To identify, delete, and replace negative self concepts and beliefs, we need to access the subconscious. We need to deal with the difficulty where it resides.

When Cognitive or other talk therapies fail, or are only helpful in a surface kind of way, it is usually because people are dealing only with the conscious mind. If the client has a consciously aware "Aha!", a truth revelation, and the problem does not go away, there are about two reasons that happens. For example, there was an "Aha!" that the thought of too much responsibility, the amount recently assumed, freaked the person out. There was a part of that individual that did not want any more responsibility than there was before. A decision needed to follow the surfaced awareness or the anxiety would not abate. The decision needs to be, after full consideration of the pros and cons, to unequivocally accept fault as well as accolades and their consequences. In other words, the decision needed to be an embrace of the total concept of responsibility. Subconscious resolution of such a matter is far easier, faster and more comprehensive than talk therapy can provide.

There are five ways to access the subconscious:
1. "Trancing out," as for example when we find ourselves staring into space,

not blinking (the "trancing out," in this case, ends when we blink)
2. Trauma
3. A state of anxiety or fear that may not reach the intensity of trauma
4. Sodium pentothal, or others in the "truth serum" family of drugs
5. Hypnosis

Of these, hypnosis is the most easily controlled. Hypnosis is not a cure in and of itself, but a key. It is simply a way to open the door and access the subconscious, where thorough healing can take place. Hypnosis is a highly effective, highly efficient way to bypass the critical faculty of the conscious mind, with its propensity to say, "Yeah, but..." and then it may proceed to undermine change and healing.

There are several ways to become hypnotized. Especially at the beginning, there is comfort to the client in the use of the Progressive Relaxation form of induction. It does not have a surreal aspect to it. Later, other methods such as the Eye Roll technique might be used. With the Progressive Relaxation induction, people are familiar with the process of suggesting from one part of the body to the next to relax that part. I explain that even if they are feeling anxious inside, body parts can be relaxed independently of that fact.

During the induction, the door opens to the marvelous subconscious depository that contains a vast wealth of data to be mined using a variety of hypnoanalytic techniques. Hypnosis is the key that opens the door to one's truth seeking journey. Under hypnosis, we gain access to those thousands of self concepts and beliefs that make each of us, quite uniquely, who we are. Even identical twins become different personalities (Harris, 2006). As but one example, imagine the birthing process. Whether the twins come down the birth canal or are removed by C - Section, one is identified as first to arrive and the other as second. In our culture, much meaning is attached to being first or second. They are already, thereby, on a different path of accumulating relevant self concepts and beliefs about themselves that will then become a constellation around the meaning of being first or of being second.

There are a variety of hypnoanalytic techniques with which to mine the data necessary to foster a thoroughgoing healing experience. One of those techniques is called age regression. The subconscious is instructed to seek the most critical the most relevant memory to the problem being addressed. The awareness warehouse is open and the subconscious, uncritically, without evaluation follows the suggestion. It brings to conscious awareness the needed memory.

In much keener detail, the subconscious can "remember" the event with greater clarity and depth of actual emotion much more so than the conscious mind can, assuming the conscious mind recollects that particular memory at all. Then, in fleshing out the memory with the client, the most important question to ask is, "How did what you just describe make you feel?" How a person "felt" in that trauma memory becomes some of their troublesome self concepts that foster their problems in the now. Taking word for word notes, this wealth of data is recorded.

Examples of this phenomenon of fleshing out feelings to identify self concepts and beliefs are these. A person may say, "I feel weak." And that you were made to feel weak, how did that make you feel? *"Angry," "helpless,"* might be additional felt reactions. Preceding further, what did you do with your angry feelings? The response: "They are still there. There was *nothing I could do about them.*" How do you manage such angry feelings today? "By *smoking*, it helps by allowing me to suck my angry feelings down."

The client has now provided a lot of information, though not all that is necessary, with which to begin changing the self concept smoker to non smoker, for example. In addition, it is clear that a trauma is in need of being worked through. Then too the anger that is residing in the body contributing to dis-ease requires therapeutic discharge and removal.

Because of such a thoroughgoing process, remember the way I was brought so quickly to eating with control—and why the capacity to eat with control has stayed with me all these years? The door to my subconscious was opened, the relevant trauma instigated by my Uncle identified, its attendant emotions and negative reactive decisions fleshed out and then in the healing phase psychotherapeutic strategies such as Cognitive Therapy and Transactional Analysis were brought into play. We dealt with my "eating out of control" *where it lived.* My subconscious was brought into harmony with my conscious desire to eat with better self control.

During this interactive type of hypnosis, people tend to float among alpha, beta, and theta states. Core Healing works at any of these levels. Wherever people gravitate is fine.

Bottom line, comprehensive healing work must occur at the subconscious level—and hypnosis is the best, most practical way to access the subconscious.

Hypnosis gives us fuller use of everything people know and have experienced, even things they may not realize they know. It allows the therapist to pinpoint precisely the negative self concepts and beliefs and other troublesome data that are causing a problem—rather than guessing what they might be—and to affect the healing at the level where, uncritically, it will be accepted and actualized .

We have taken an overview of Core Healing, and explored the conscious and subconscious minds. Let's look further now at how self concepts and beliefs become imprinted on the subconscious, and how we become who we are.

Chapter 3

HOW WE BECOME WHO WE ARE
(And How Dis-Ease Develops)

How do we get to be who we are? Why do we behave as we do? Why do some of us get depressed, and others overeat or starve ourselves? Why do some people have low self esteem, while others succumb to rage? Why do some people find it so difficult to quit smoking, while others do not? How does an anxiety disorder develop? Why do we start feeling unlovable?

This chapter addresses those questions. Moreover, in general terms, it discusses the roots of such dis-eases as: depression, anxiety, stress, substance abuse, eating disorders (obesity, anorexia, bulimia), purposelessness, unhealthy attractions, rage, physical problems, and unhealthy habits. Part 2 of this book explores each of the foregoing dis-eases in depth.

We have seen that the subconscious is a library or storehouse for the negative self concepts and beliefs that cause dis-ease. (Positive self concepts and beliefs are also stored, of course, but our focus will be on the negatives because we are talking about healing.) This chapter is about how those negative self concepts and beliefs get into the storehouse, and how they shape our personalities and our lives.

FAULTY THINKING: THE ROOT OF PROBLEMS

Unless we get to the root of a problem, with all its tentacles, we cannot solve it. Core Healing is about getting to the very bottom of the all of what stresses and distresses us, so that we can feel whole and become the people we have the wonderful potential to be.

After working at a core level with hundreds of clients over twenty years, I believe that most, if not all, human problems are the result of faulty thinking (or "stinkin' thinkin'," as some say) many in the form of fear based negative self concepts and beliefs. Clients, especially those who had been prone to doing anxiety and major worry, can reinfect their subconscious with negatives while in a state of fear. So they need to be taught to get into a new habit based on an absolute vigilance to avert stickin' thinkin'. Positive self statements must be at the ready under any circumstance of felt fear regardless of degree. When fear is present, access to the subconscious is immediate. It is a reaction of self protective vigilance and activates the "computer center" for "appropriate" response. So, self statements at the ready are statements like: "I'll work this out," "everything will be okay," "I can handle this," "I'm good at getting myself out of a tight spot," "I'm not dying, I am fine," etc. Like at the OK Corral, one must be ready with a six shooter loaded with the bullets of positive self statements. Fear arises. Practiced and ready, the individual must whip out this weapon to shoot down the fear that was produced in any given situation. The memorized and rehearsed phrases must *always* be at the ready. Bam, bam....the negatives are blasted away and calm prevails. A person can get that good at it.

Our beliefs determine what we think, what we feel, and what we perceive. This is why two people may witness the same event, but give dramatically different descriptions of what happened. Suppose Ann and Gerry see a red car rear-end a blue car. If Ann believes we should all live within the letter of the law and be our brothers' keepers, she might say, "The red car was going too fast and just slammed into him. She was talking on her cell phone and not paying attention. It was her fault." Gerry might believe that nobody should impede another person's progress through life—and if they do, they deserve what they get. His report on the accident might be, "The blue car just screeched to a halt in front of the red car with no warning! He put himself in the way. It was his fault."

My work tends to suggest that our thoughts and beliefs can actually influence our physiology—perhaps even our DNA, which we now know is mutable. We saw in Chapter 2 how emotions generated by negative beliefs can affect brain chemistry. People often ask about depression and brain chemicals, "Was it the chicken or the egg that came first?" Did the depressive thoughts cause the level of the brain's feel good chemical to lessen? Or, did the make up of the individual provide lower levels of the feel good chemical therefore causing the person to be depressed. Because Cognitive Behavioral Therapy combined with mindfulness has been shown to be better than drugs at curing depression (Begley, 2007), then we might choose to presume that negative self concepts and beliefs are the agent of lowered levels of the feel good chemical.

Core Healing, which incorporates aspects of the above referenced approaches to successful therapy, can cause clients to feel overdosed on their psychotropic medications. Clients are urged to be aware of that fact and to report when that feeling results from our work. Then, under the care of their prescribing physician, they are titrated, brought down gradually, from the drug(s) prescribed. If, during this process of titration, a symptom surfaces, the client is given priority access to further therapy to remove the source of the symptom so that the stepping down may comfortably continue. This suggests that the brain's chemicals are able to return to normal once there are no negative thoughts and beliefs creating a lowering effect. Life can then move forward with a wonderful sense of self control.

Our self concepts and beliefs determine our path through life. How strongly they influence us depends on their number and intensity. The direction in which they lead us depends on whether they are neutral, positive, or negative. When we include neutral and positive self concepts and beliefs in the equation, we are talking about *millions* of pieces of information. We have beliefs about everything from the nature of the universe to how a blade of grass grows. We don't usually pause to reflect on our beliefs—and even when we do, it is usually on our *conscious* beliefs. The strength of Core Healing is that it takes us beyond those conscious beliefs to the information in the subconscious that, literally, creates our lives and makes us who we are.

HOW WE BECOME WHO WE ARE

How do we acquire all these negative self concepts and beliefs? Remember that they are stored in the subconscious. That means that the door to the subconscious must be open in order for them to enter.

We saw in the last chapter that there are five ways to access the subconscious:
1. Trancing out," as but one example when we find ourselves staring into space, not blinking (the "trancing out" ends when we blink)
2. Trauma
3. A state of anxiety or fear that may not reach the intensity of trauma
4. Sodium pentothal, or others in the "truth serum" family of drugs
5. Hypnosis

The first three are fairly common occurrences, and they are the primary ways that our subconscious opens to the development of self concepts and beliefs, whether they be positive or more usually negative, especially when traumatized or fearful.

It was once thought that at conception we were a *tabula rasa*, an erased or clean slate. Now, research suggests, that we are wired with a temperament, a nature versus nurture issue. From a self preservation standpoint, for example, we are wary creatures which assuredly affects our personalities. How wary an individual can depend upon nature. Assuredly, nonetheless, an individual can be sensitized to a heightened level of wariness as a result of circumstance, in other words the nurture factor. The womb itself is, of course, an environment that can nurture for the better or for the detriment of an individual. It can be a calm and loving or turbulent and anxiety producing milieu.

In the womb, we can begin "collecting" subconsciously stored self concepts and beliefs, and we continue until the day we die. These self concepts can be reinforced or not, and, if not, they are not as likely to impact the behavior or the emotions of the individual over the course of a lifetime.

Here is one example of how self concept development works. Suppose that, at age four, Sally gets introduced to her five year old cousin, Tommy. He pushes her. She falls down and scrapes her elbow. In her state of anxiety and fear, several negative self concepts and beliefs get imprinted on her subconscious. Some of them may be suggested by other negatives that are already in place, even at her young age. The ones that get stored in Sally's subconscious that day might be:

- "Strange boys are dangerous."
- "Boys want to hurt me."
- "Strangers are out to get you."
- "I am unlovable."
- "I deserve to be hurt."
- "I can't stand up for myself when someone pushes me."

In later life, these negatives might manifest as shyness, inappropriate physical fears, difficulty in relationships with men, or any number of other conditions that express those particular beliefs.

Once a negative belief has been stored in the subconscious, it begins to shape how we think, act, and what we attract into our lives. When a sight, sound, smell, emotion, similar situation, or *anything* triggers that self concept or belief, we act on it as if it were absolutely true—even when our conscious mind tells us that it is definitely not true. It doesn't matter how many times Sally's mother or aunt might tell her, "Tommy didn't push you. He was falling himself, and accidentally bumped into you." What matters is not what happened, but what we think happened at the moment of the incident and what we decided as a result. It doesn't matter that Tommy didn't really push Sally; what matters is that she *thought* he pushed her and that her subconscious imprinted beliefs based on that interpretation.

When we adopt a negative self concept or belief, we are rarely aware that we have done so. Nor are we usually aware when these negatives get triggered by people, events, or perceptions in our present lives. Only when we begin to question our behavior and ask why we act the way we do, and when we are open to discovering the truth, will we be willing to adventure beneath the surface and find out what is really going on.

Sharon was willing to explore. She had dated a series of men who left her, or who were married, or emotionally distant, or gay, or in some other way unavailable for the kind of physical and emotional intimacy she craved. She had the courage to admit, "There's only one common element in all these relationships—me!" Under hypnosis, Sharon saw why it was inevitable that she would be attracted to these kinds of men. Her father traveled for his work and was distracted when he did spend time at home. Under hypnosis, she relived an incident that occurred when she was four. Her father had arrived home from a business trip and brushed her mother aside with, "Leave me alone. I need some peace and quiet."

In our session, Sharon experienced the same emotions she had experienced that day—fear and anxiety that she or her mother had done something wrong and might be abandoned—and saw clearly how she had adopted beliefs that "Husbands are never home," "Men don't like to be bothered," and "Men aren't available emotionally even when their bodies are in the room," which is a form of abandonment. In the remainder of the Core Healing process, she was able to dissolve those negative beliefs and replace them with, "I can attract men who are available, and who want to be emotionally and physically intimate." That helped her make choices based on what she truly wanted, rather than what her subconscious had decided she deserved on one particular day when she was four.

What we do, say, and think—the things that make us who we are—are simply the automatic responses of our subconscious self concepts and beliefs to external stimuli. Our computer mind, the subconscious, is simply reacting to one stimulus after another, instantaneously pulling from its library of self concepts the ones that produce a relevant response. The response may be desirable or not, based on the self concepts that generated it.

CONSTELLATIONS

As we go through life, we acquire more and more self concepts and beliefs. Each one tends to be based on, and to support, those that are already in place. I call these groups of reinforcing self concepts and beliefs "constellations." Constellations can also be fluid. Their composition can reformulate based on a given stimulus.

Early on, we develop propensity for either positive or negative beliefs, depending on whether we started out with more positives or more negatives. If we start out with a preponderance of positive self concepts and beliefs—"I am lovable," "I can trust myself and others," "I am competent and able"—we are more likely to collect more positives that reinforce our earlier ones, and thus to have an easier time in life. If we begin with a preponderance of negatives—"I deserve to be abandoned," "I deserve to be punished," "I come second in life," "I'm not good enough"—we tend to accumulate more negatives and to have a more difficult time.

Gathering beliefs that reinforce these basic, key beliefs is a natural process. If I come into the world with a belief that "I must be bad," then I may have a tendency to act badly. That increases my chances of being involved in negative events that reinforce the belief that "I must be bad." Eventually, I may gather a constellation of hundreds of beliefs that reinforce that unfortunate original one.

Whether or not subsequent events actually do reinforce the original beliefs, we tend to *interpret* them that way—and that is all that matters. The original self concepts and beliefs that were imprinted on Sally's subconscious when Tommy "pushed" her attracted a constellation of beliefs that included, as she went through life, "I can't trust anybody," "People are just out to hurt me," and "Men are rough and violent." Obviously, there was evidence in Sally's life for the opposites of these new beliefs as well. Certainly there was somebody she could trust. All people were not out to hurt her. All men are not rough and violent. But Sally didn't see that. Her early negative beliefs formed her ground of being, the way she approached life. It was from that point of view that she saw the events around her, and so what she saw reinforced those beliefs.

NEGATIVE REACTIVE DECISIONS

Many of our self concepts and beliefs are the result of negative reactive decisions, knee-jerk responses to events or conditions. My Uncle chided me for being fat. My juvenile response? I'll eat what I want, whenever I want and however much I want. He can't stop me. Food is a key arena where a child can be in control. The goal is not to create, unwittingly as my Uncle did, a set up for an immature, rebellious reactive decision. (This reactive decision is rampant among obese individuals.)

Negative reactive decisions are numerous and varied. One of my clients, Helen, had been thin all her life. But when she got married, she started gaining weight. After four years of marriage, she had gained about forty pounds. She came to me because she just couldn't seem to lose it. She had been raised to believe that after you were married, you shouldn't flirt with other men. Before she was married, Helen had been very coquettish and playful sexually. She loved flirting and gathering all the men around her at parties. The negative reactive decision she made in order to stay true to her standards was: "I'll get fat, and then the guys won't respond to my flirting." It was her way to stay safe, but it was hurting her in other areas, including her health. When she realized, under hypnosis, what she had strategized, we could delete that negative belief and replace it with, "I can be thin, healthy, attractive <u>and</u> faithful," or "I don't choose to see being flirtatious as fun. Having the faithful attention of my husband is *much* more fun."

NO TWO ARE ALIKE   (Harris, 2006)

The process of accumulating self concepts and beliefs is highly individual. It is dictated by our specific circumstances, moment to moment, by how we respond to those circumstances, and by the self concepts and beliefs that are already in place. This is why no two people are alike—not even identical twins, as mentioned earlier. No two individuals, no matter how similar their genetics, have exactly the same set of events, circumstances, interactions, and reactions. Therefore, no two individuals have the same set of self concepts and beliefs. Therefore, no two individuals have exactly the same personality.

Imagine two soldiers on a battlefield. Bullets are zooming over their heads. It is a terrifying situation, the ultimate "fight or flight" stimulus. The situation is exactly the same for these two men, but their reactions are entirely different. The first solder tries not to run, but he does. His ideas about courage and valor are trumped by a preponderance of self concepts and beliefs that support running. The second soldier remains and fights even harder, the result of a different set of self concepts and beliefs. The stimulus is the same. Both are threatened with death. But because their self concepts and beliefs are different, their responses are different.

Similarly, in such trauma events as produced by war, one's constellations of self concepts and beliefs will either inoculate a person from the affects of witnessing horrifying events, or they will produce a post traumatic stress reaction.

John came to me with a post traumatic stress reaction that was manifesting as withdrawal from life to the confines of his home. In his senior year at college, he worked nights at a pizza place. Just at closing time, two ski masked people with guns came in to rob the store. One of them forced my client to stand in a corner as he kept a gun to his head. When John came to me for therapy, he reported that the others showed no ill affect from the trauma, just him. That became the issue. Why him? Clearing out his relevant negative self concepts and beliefs allowed John to return to school.

HOW OUR PERSONALITIES DEVELOP

Part of Core Healing's effectiveness comes from the following model of personality development. In order to systematically identify, delete, and replace negative self concepts and beliefs, we need to know how our personalities develop from fetus to senior citizen. Here is a brief outline.

Gestation

At conception, as mentioned earlier, we begin our physical development that seems to be part and parcel in the development of aspects of temperament. Based upon my work, I can't help but wonder if the environment that a mother provides as a result of her thought processes and resulting emotion(s) affects and effects the development of a fetus' temperament including the third trimester surge of opposite sex hormone which is now attributed to the development of homosexual conduct.

At six weeks into gestation, the brain is formed. Its neural network is in a state of rapid growth and expansion. At four months, the fetus can pick up vibrations—both physical and emotional.

On a purely physical level, the amniotic fluid is always moving as the mother and baby move. We know that amniotic fluid carries physical vibrations, and that these vibrations have differing characters. If you simply stick your finger in water, for example, the water ripples out and creates one kind of vibration. If you twirl your finger and churn the water, you create a different *quality* of vibration. One is smooth, the other is more turbulent. Even voice sounds cause vibrations in the amniotic fluid. This is one reason obstetricians are now recommending that prospective parents play classical music and talk lovingly to the mother's belly during pregnancy. It seems that emotional vibrations are carried in these ways, and that the fetus can sense without words or conscious awareness the emotional signature of what is happening outside the womb.

On the subconscious level, these movements and vibrations suggest to the fetus how hospitable or inhospitable the environment is. Obviously, the baby has no language to translate "felt senses" into words, but "feeling" data of consequence is imprinted into the subconscious: being wanted or not wanted, loved or not loved, at ease or stressed, worthy or unworthy of existing, good enough or not, secure or insecure about survival. One very common "felt sense" is anxiety, perhaps because most mothers generate some anxiety about pregnancy and birth, regardless of how much they do, or do not, want the baby. The fetus picks up these vibrations.

Quite often, anxiety disorder has its roots in the womb. Many of my clients who have experienced being back in the womb under hypnotic regression say that they felt anxious, frightened, trapped, or unwanted. Because the subconscious governs physiology, some of those who felt particularly unwanted had breech or otherwise difficult or late births—a reflection of their reluctance to enter an inhospitable world.

When people say, "I've been a nervous person all my life," the roots of that anxiety are often in the womb. The fetus absorbs the mother's anxiety, which triggers the "fight or flight" response. Since there isn't much a fetus can do about fighting or "flighting" while in the womb other than perhaps abort, the anxiety stays in place and translates into a generalized nervousness or insecurity. After the birth, these babies are often described as "colicky," agitated, or nervous. As children, they can develop hyper vigilance, a hypersensitive response to anything that might seem remotely threatening to their survival or well being.

The situation for the fetus is exacerbated when the mother has thoughts like:
- "I can't afford this."
- "My boyfriend and I are having trouble, and I don't think this relationship is going to work out."
- "What am I going to do? We can't afford this baby, and my religion won't let me have an abortion."
- "I don't really want this kid."

The fetus picks up these vibrations, and makes black-or-white evaluations. Some self concepts and beliefs that might be imprinted, based on the above, are: "I am a problem. I shouldn't exist," "I must deserve to be abandoned," "I deserve to be killed," and "I'm not desirable." When people relive these memories and "felt senses" as adults, they can put words to what was happening. The beliefs can then be deleted and replaced, and the trauma desensitized, even many years after the events occurred.

Some negative self concepts and beliefs often picked up in the womb are:
- "I am not wanted."
- "I shouldn't exist."
- "I'm anxious."
- "I'm sad."
- "I must be no good."
- "I'm scared to come into the world."
- "I deserve to be abandoned."

Some positives that also occur frequently, and that can help produce contented infants are:
- "It's relaxed in here. This is nice."
- "I am wanted."
- "I feel loved."
- "My parents are happy to have me."

Sadly for Carlo, when his problem took him back to his experience of being in the womb, he said he felt frantic and wanted to throw up. Of course, a fetus cannot vomit, but that was the feeling he had. His mother had been a smoker, and Carlo was being nauseated by the toxicity of the smoke. The feeling of being nauseous, but unable to throw up, created a panic reaction. What got imprinted in Carlo's subconscious was a generalized sense of significant anxiety, which he brought with him into life outside the womb and which was only alleviated when he could identify, delete, and replace his trapped feelings with a sense of ease and serenity that result from the obvious reality that he was no longer trapped.

The birthing experience itself has the potential to be fraught with trauma. It is another opportunity to imprint positive or negative self concepts and beliefs. How the birth is handled, and how it is perceived by the newly born, can result in a multitude of reactions ranging from "This world is a cold, blindingly light, and terrible place" to "Coming into this world is welcoming, warm, and cozy."

Events can also occur after the birth that threaten the baby's sense of well being and security. These threats are experienced sensually (by touch, sight, smell, sound, taste, and general "sense of things") and imprinted on the subconscious. As language develops, words and thoughts capture the felt senses and become self concepts or beliefs. For example, suppose a mother dies in childbirth. The father is distraught. There is no family to help him. He feels at a total loss to be a parent on his own, and decides to put the baby up for adoption. Adoptive parents are found. From the adult viewpoint, everything is being done with great consideration. The newborn is being cared for, and everything is going well. But the newborn may experience these events very differently—as a catastrophe. The infant is panicked, literally "scared to death" that she will not survive without a mother or father, and feels trapped in her dependency. The infant is all "felt senses," and feels abandoned, but more than that, freaked out scared and in a primal way. She has no larger world view, no language or logic, no maturity to help her through this time.

Children's minds tend to generalize from the specific to the general, from one experience to all of life. If their initial perceptions are positive, then they tend to meet the world with positive expectations, and therefore receive positive impressions. It's another way to view the law of attraction. (Byrne, 2006) If the initial perceptions are negative, they can tend to look at life "through a glass darkly." Gradually, children build larger and larger constellations of self concepts and beliefs that are either positive or negative or stressfully competitive. An example of the latter case: "I'm dumb...but I know I'm smart."

Infancy

Two of the biggest challenges in infancy are the fear of being alone, and the fear of being abandoned. Obviously, these two fears intertwine—and both translate into the fear of dying.

Infants are helpless. If they are left entirely alone, with no one to feed or care for them, they do die—and on some level, they know it. Since they don't yet have language, we can't explain to them that we are only going away for a few minutes or a few hours. Infants cannot understand that their parents are coming back, or that they have seen to all the infant's needs in their absence. All infants know is that the people on whom they depend for survival have left.

Parents do the best they can, but they cannot possibly be there for infants 24/7. Aside from the natural needs of sleeping, going to the bathroom, and bathing, all kinds of intrusions and circumstances demand the parents' attention. The phone rings. Another child needs help. It is virtually impossible to avoid leaving an infant in the safety of the crib for at least short periods of time.

Suppose the mother is fixing dinner with her infant in a crib nearby. A neighbor pounds on the door and pleads hysterically, "My husband just fell down. I think he's had a heart attack. Can you please come help me?" The mother looks at the infant, and figures he'll be safe while she leaves and helps her neighbor for two minutes. But she winds up being gone a little longer than she expected, and the infant goes into a state of panic. He is dependant on her for survival, and she has left him. He has no way of knowing where she went, why, or when she will be back. His "felt sense" tells him, "I am abandoned, and I'm going to die."

If this experience happens just once, then other, more positive experiences may mitigate it. But if it happens often, for long periods of time, if his needs have not been met just prior to the parent leaving, or if his parents' reaction to his crying is guilt or anger, then he may literally grow up being "scared to death" of being alone. Infants with a base of positive self concepts, who have felt welcomed, happy, loved, and secure are likely to do better with being left alone—barring any associated trauma, like a fire—than infants who already feel a little tenuous.

Adopted infants are particularly susceptible to the *in utero* into infancy development of negative self concepts and beliefs. Not only are they more likely to encounter fear, anger, panic, helplessness, and a general sense of not being wanted or loved in utero, but they are also subject to feeling abandoned and left in the time between birth and adoption. This can be a time of stark terror that results in feelings of being not good enough, of deserving to be punished, of being unlovable, and especially of being abandoned. A debilitating belief that "I don't deserve to be taken care of" ensues. In adulthood, that becomes spending money recklessly, being fat, depressed, etc.

Adoptive parents often say, "I don't know what I did, but my kid is acting way out of control. This kid is off the wall." Not all adoptive children are a handful, but many are. They have had more opportunity than most infants to acquire negative self concepts and beliefs, both *in utero* and immediately after birth.

Childhood

In childhood, the process of accumulating self concepts and beliefs continues. Children have language, and they are starting to move out into the world. They notice that they have bodies. ("I have the body of a girl" or "I have the body of a boy.") They start to acquire a whole new set of labels. ("I am a good girl," "I am a good reader," "I'm stupid at school.") They begin to notice cultural attributes. ("I belong to a middle class family.") They learn about race. ("I am white," "I am Latino," "I am African-American.") They may be exposed to religion and develop beliefs. ("Ethics are important," "God does/does not love me.")

Negative self concepts and beliefs that are frequently acquired in childhood are:
- "I'm shy."
- "I'm stupid."
- "I'm unattractive."
- "I'm fat."
- "I'm bad."
- "I'm a loser."
- "I can't let myself get angry."
- "I'm not good enough/smart enough/thin enough."
- "I'm unlovable."
- "I don't deserve to be loved unconditionally."
- "I must deserve to be abandoned."

Some of these beliefs simply reinforce negative self concepts and beliefs from infancy. Others may be reactions to new situations like divorce or the mother going back to work. Still others may rise out of going to school and having experiences like not being picked for the team until last or getting negative academic feedback. This is often how "I'm stupid" gets started or reinforced—and it is an extremely common self concept. Most of us have an intense fear of doing or saying something that might be considered stupid. Even the brightest adults often say, "I know I'm intelligent, but there is a part of me that thinks of myself as stupid." We will go to great lengths not to appear dumb or stupid, doing whatever we can to avoid the kind of ridicule, embarrassment and humiliation we were made to feel as a "stupid" child—either at school or by shaming parents.

Another fear that many of us develop in childhood is the fear of anger. Anger can be frightening to witness, and some children develop a belief that they must avoid getting angry, or being around anger, at any price. This might result in, "I'll give in rather than upset others," or "I can never get angry, because I can't trust myself not to hurt someone."

But children also notice the power that anger gives the person who wields it. In a home where anger is used by parents to control children, children may be forced into one of three negative options:

- They rebel.
- They comply and lose their spirit.
- They learn to use anger in the same way their parents do.

They learn that they can use anger to intimidate or control others, and that doing so can alleviate some of their own fear. Once they have used anger successfully to control or intimidate, either on the playground or at home with their siblings, the self concept is born: "I am a person who enjoys feeling the power of controlling others with my anger."

This self concept is catalogued in the subconscious under the heading of "Methods for Controlling Others" with a cross reference to "Temper Inducing Situations." These catalogued references are now available for retrieval as an "appropriate" reaction to fear, or to feeling out of control. The price includes resentment, smoldering rage, volcanic eruptions, and a condition in which the child, and later the adult, is actually controlled by people and situations outside himself. He *has* to react with anger to certain kinds of people and situations because of the propelling self concepts and beliefs.

Source of control is a critical factor in this work. Are we controlled by people and situations outside ourselves, or by substances, or can we choose appropriate responses and resources? The whole point of freeing ourselves of negative self concepts and beliefs is to regain the power to choose wisely, and to keep the source of control within ourselves. That lets us be ourselves, actualize our potential, and contribute to life. If we abdicate the source of control to others through ignorance, fear and/or naivete, we lose that freedom. Autocrats who demand blind obedience, unprincipled plutocrats, and, theocracies are major threats to our core beings, to our loss of autonomy. Moreover, if we imitate others in imagining that substances will provide control over discomforting feelings, ironically, we lose control. Finally, if we seek to control others, we lose control of our own essence, our own meaning.

An anger filled home may produce two quite different children Some examples are one might be pacific, the other a bully, one may be timid another fiery. It depends on prior accumulated self concepts and beliefs. Children raised in the same house, by the same parents, can be dramatically different from one another. Again, no two are alike. Some of the many factors involved are:

- The parents are at different stages of life, and different ages, when the different children are born.
- Birth order, and the presence or absence of other siblings, has an impact. The parents themselves gain experience with each successive child, which can work to the good or to the detriment of the younger siblings— depending on the nature of their parents' experience. If the parents have learned that anger is a good way to keep the kids in line, it may work to their detriment. If the parents have learned to give positive reinforcement, the younger children may have an easier time.
- The sex of the child and what being a boy means to a child or what being a girl means can affect the self concepts that develop. For varying reasons, each of us is simply a uniquely evolving person, with a unique set of circumstances and reactions.

Shyness

One of the most powerful negative self concepts that often develops during childhood is *shyness*. Suppose Allen is five when his mother opens the door to greet her friend. To Allen, this woman is a stranger—and very large. (I often think the story of how shyness develops should be called "In the Land of the Giants.") Our basic animal instincts make us wary in the presence of people and things that are bigger than we are and might be dangerous. This caution is a natural protective device. Allen hides behind his mother, who says, "Oh, Allen, don't be shy. Mrs. Smith is Mommy's *friend*!"

Because he is frightened, Allen's subconscious mind is available. He is immediately imprinted with the belief that he is a shy person, and also that there is something shameful about being shy. His self concept of "I am shy" will have definitions attached to it as he proceeds through life. Those definitions wil effect his degree of introversion. Shyness not only makes social situations more difficult, but is a significant contributing factor in many types of substance abuse.

Alcohol, for example, lowers one's inhibitions. The "shy" young adult is in a bind. He fears being alone but is scared of people, as the word shy suggests. Alcohol greases the wheel to deal with those fears. The young person can then go out, party and not be alone.

The amount of alcohol consumed seems directly proportional to the amount of fear (and pain) that an individual feels. That about half of college students today are binge drinking can only suggest just how freaked out scared they are, and in what terrible emotional pain they must find themselves, whether or not they are consciously aware of how they actually feel. Binging, whatever form it takes, whether with drugs, alcohol, food, spending, sex, etc. what is being dealt with at core is *primal* fear, internally generated, stark terror. Primal fear is in itself *painful*.

Prevention

What can parents do to give their children the best possible chance to grow up with more positive than negative self concepts and beliefs? It is actually very simple. Children tend to believe what their parents tell them, quite literally. Parents who want their children to have positive experiences avoid negative name-calling like "stupid," "dumb," "bad boy," and "loser." Remember, children think from the specific to the general. When you say, "Bad boy," you may be talking about him not picking up his toys—but he may be hearing that he is a bad person.

Other phrases that stick with us are ones like:
- "You'll never amount to anything."
- "Why can't you be like....?"

- "What's the matter with you? You never get it right."
- "Who could ever love a kid like you?"
- "You disgust me. Get out of my face."
- "What you've done is unforgivable."

Instead, get into the habit of using phrases that reinforce children's positive self concepts and that help them think of themselves in positive ways. Try using nurturing, but *earned* phrases like:

- "Even though you didn't quite get it right yet, based on past experience, you will."
- "You're improving."
- "I am so proud of you and how you stick with it."
- "That was a thoughtful thing you just did."
- "You're getting smarter every day." (Be specific.)
- "Helping that little girl from Guatemala sew doll clothes is a wonderful way to use one of your talents."
- "I am angry with what you said just now because it seems unfair to judge me without knowing the whole story—but knowing you as I do, I know you will be open to listening to the rest of what I have to say."

Giving feedback in context that is genuine, respectful, positive, and routine will not only remove any potential for feeling it is hokum but will limit the potential for a false sense of self esteem.

The Teen Years

The teen years can be a tortured time, with anxiety and fear opening the subconscious to a multitude of new negative self concepts. This is an awkward time by any standards, awash with words like "pimple face," "geek," "nerd," "fag," "weirdo," "freak," and all the other ugly words that teens use to make their peers miserable...most likely as miserably as they feel about themselves. That we accept such unkind conduct as, "it's just the way kids are" is unfair to them. It is not a genetic defect. Being mean to each other is simply that.

Teens who have accumulated large constellations of negative self concepts and beliefs in childhood are particularly vulnerable. Some of the negatives that tend to arise or be reinforced during the teenage years are:

- "I'm bad."

- "I'm dumb."
- "I'm evil."
- "I'm ugly."
- "I'm inferior."
- "I'm a freak."
- "I might be, or I am a queer."

Sometimes teens withdraw to their rooms, which they turn into caves with their own music and games, and pictures of their heroes. Fear and rage are common, as most parents of teens are well aware—whether the teens act out in violent ways, or are more prone to fear and paralysis.

The teen years are also when eating disorders often start to manifest. People tend to hide in their fat, and the teen years are often a time when we want to hide. Fat is also a form of punishment and/or self abandonment, and a way to protect ourselves from being approached sexually. By the teen years, obese children's eating-related negative self concepts and beliefs are usually firmly entrenched. Some of these are:

- "I'm fat and I can't help it."
- "The more I eat, the better it makes my parents feel." (These are members of the Clean Plate Club.)
- "Eating volumes of food is how you are supposed to eat."
- "I deserve to be humiliated and in pain for being a fat child."
- "I deserve to be rejected."
- "I am unlovable as I am."
- "I am lazy."

Anorexia and bulimia can also surface in the teen years, with their own sets of negative self concepts and beliefs which we discuss in Chapter 11.

Adulthood

Personality development continues into adulthood, both reinforcing old self concepts and acquiring new ones. Their world of experience broadens. Now we are dealing with more adult experiences, but the process is the same. The door to the subconscious opens—usually as a result of fear, trauma, anxiety, or simply "trancing out"—and the negative self concept or belief gets imprinted.

We may start to think of ourselves as fragile, depressed, anxious, accident prone, lousy lovers, unfaithful, or failures. The profession we choose may also carry self concepts that we adopt. Doctors may think of themselves as intelligent but driven. An artist might think of herself as anti-social or flighty. A computer programmer might develop the self concept of being obsessive or nerdy. The older we get, the more opportunities we have had to acquire self concepts and beliefs.

Again, these can be positive or negative, severe or light. Often the process is subtle. As adults, we continue with one of our primary goals/beliefs which is to avoid pain. When avoiding pain is packaged with the ancillary belief, *at all costs*, trouble will arise. We are *not taught strategic pain management*. When avoiding the pain of one experience, people must be keenly aware not to create a pain management system that produces a whole other kind of pain. So, suppose we experience a painful ending to a romantic relationship. Unwittingly, in that moment of fear and emotional trauma, or even just while trancing out as we walk or drive, we might "suggest" to our subconscious an idea to avert pain forever: "I'll never fall in love again." Another negative reactive self concept might be: "I don't know if I could pull myself out (of that kind of pain) again." And yet another, "I'm just going to be a playboy."

Once those self concepts are in place, walls go up. By not consciously thinking through our plans for protecting ourselves, by not exploring the consequences of our choices, we actually create whole *new sources of pain*. As a result of our hastily derived decision, we may not have the pain of a failed relationship again, but we experience the pain of isolation, loneliness, shallow relationships, or perhaps gaining weight to protect ourselves from intimacy.

Of course, positive self concepts and beliefs can be imprinted as well. A self concept can change instantaneously if someone, either in a state of fear or while trancing out, starts thinking along these lines: "Smoking is bad. I don't enjoy it. It's harming me and I don't deserve to be harmed. I'm not going to be a smoker anymore." That person may just have changed his or her self concept into that of a non-smoker, if there were no consequential negative self concepts to block the implementation.

The process of self concept development is continuous and usually without our conscious knowledge. When he was in his twenties, Alex attended the funeral of a close friend. As the coffin was lowered into the ground, the sun glinted off the shiny silver curve of its side. Soon after that, Alex developed a terror of flying.

Since his job involved constant travel, this was a serious matter. Under hypnosis, Alex recalled the friend's funeral, and the subconscious belief that had become imprinted: "Being inside a shiny silver curved object is death." He immediately thought of the fuselage of an airplane and realized that to enter one of them had become equated, in his subconscious, with being inside a coffin!

As adults, we often recreate the patterns of our family of origin. Where do we get our ideas about how husbands and wives are supposed to interact? Mostly, from our parents. We almost always find ourselves attracted to people with whom we can recreate the world of our original family. We wind up finding spouses, bosses, friends, lovers, and others who are like our parents and siblings—and interacting with them as we did with our family. Our self concepts and beliefs are often based primarily on that world, for better or worse. This is why we often hear people say, "I married my father," or "My boss is just like my brother!" Then, when these awarenesses dawn upon us, self concepts can develop like "I'll never get married again," or "I don't want another wife like my mother."

The Senior Years

At this point, quality of life issues start coming into play—and so does the fact that death is closer than it was in our early and middle years.

The danger here is living in fear, or letting new physical problems define us. We may develop aches and pains, high blood pressure or cholesterol, decreasing mental acuity, or any other of the difficulties that often accompany old age. Some people simply give up, saying, "Well, I'm old now. I can't do anything." Others subconsciously decide, "I'd better do everything I can *now*." Which road a person chooses has a lot to do with the positive or negative quality of the self concepts and beliefs that he or she has accumulated over a lifetime.

In a state of fear, fragility can be nourished. Or, we can actually use the subconscious to program for healing and rejuvenation. By recognizing negative self concepts and turning them into positives at the subconscious level, we give ourselves power over them and facilitate self healing. We don't have to let anger reside in our bones, joints, or anywhere else where they might do mischief. Remember: "Heal the mind, the body follows."

LABELS

Labeling the conditions that rise out of our negative self concepts and beliefs can strengthen those beliefs, and even create new ones. It is difficult to avoid using words like "depression," "anxiety disorder," "addict," and "eating disorder"—but when people define themselves as "a depressed person" or "an addict," the self concept gets more deeply embedded and can even become a way of life. They can become their labels.

For instance, an "anxious person" or "anxiety-disordered person" may begin to act even more "anxiety-disordered." Depending on how this condition is defined, she may act even more nervous, fidgety, inattentive, or unfocused. She may bite her nails, curl her fingers around in her hair, or tap her foot. She defines herself as an "anxious person," and her behavior naturally conforms to her ideas of what an "anxious person" does, most likely including smoking.

SECONDARY GAIN

When we talk about negative self concepts and beliefs, we also need to be aware of what is called "secondary gain." Secondary gain is *whatever we get out of having a particular problem*. Often, we believe we could not get what we want if we didn't have that particular physical or mental incapacity.

Rhonda was in a state of high anxiety when she came to see me. She was pregnant, and I could tell she had all the makings for *post partum* depression. (Anxiety that is left unchecked deepens into depression.) On a conscious level, she was thrilled about being a mother. She and her husband had all their ducks lined up. They had great jobs, they could afford the baby, they had a beautiful suburban home in Evanston (a city just north of Chicago), and both wanted to be parents. Except that, after she got pregnant, Rhonda became increasingly anxious, almost panicky—and couldn't figure out why.

It took awhile for her to look beyond the conscious mind's insistence that, "Oh, I'm ready. I can't wait. I have the bassinet, the clothes, everything!" When we accessed her subconscious mind, Rhonda saw that she was terrified of being "responsible" for the baby because she was afraid that somehow or other she might injure it. Anyone who knew Rhonda would have been surprised by this, because she acted like the most responsible, gentle person in the world. She was a dental hygienist, an upstanding citizen who paid her bills and lived an exemplary life. But subconsciously, the thought of being responsible for a baby's well being was more than she could handle.

Keep in mind that one's thoughts and beliefs can affect hormonal response as is the case for example when danger is present. Adrenalin and other fright/flight hormones charge up the body for a self protective reaction. Remembering that, let's now enter the domain of Rhonda's reality, her subconscious mind. Just about everyone knows, including Rhonda who is pregnant, that there can be a hormonal imbalance after delivery that produces a condition called Post Partum Depression. The chicken or the egg—which comes first—the fears and negative self concept and beliefs that lead to hormonal effect, or does the body in response to the pregnancy produce an imbalance? My work with Core Healing suggests that Post Partum Depression results from the conflict of opposing constellations. Post Partum Depression is a metaphor for the individual's relevant constellations being out of balance. On the one hand, the pregnant mom wants the baby. On the other hand, she fears the responsibility for the baby, especially for its security. There are those women who have a heavy duty fear of hurting the child in one way or another, either emotionally and/or physically. It depends upon the configuration of each one's constellation. We have read about some women who have become good mothers after the fears in their constellation of negatives dissipate in view of their realizing they are being good to their child. Their positive self concepts and beliefs wind up dominating and surmounting the negatives. Then, at the extreme other end, there are women whose constellation of negatives so dominate, that they literally kill their children. Change the self concepts and save the baby.

Rhonda, as a result of the deletion of her negative constellation and enhanced positive one, was free to be in harmony. The desire to have a child was now supported by a host of positive self concepts and beliefs.

THE CONSEQUENCE—AND THE HOPE

Our negative self concepts and beliefs are at the bottom of most, if not all, of our physical and psychological difficulties. As the negative constellations grow, they gain power and rob us of health, happiness, productivity, and serenity.

The good news is this: We do not have to live at the effect of those negative self concepts and beliefs, and we don't have to let them define us. None of us is immune to their effects, but knowing how they work and participating in Core Healing can minimize their impact and even eradicate them forever.

During Core Healing, we delete some 200-400 negative self concepts and beliefs and replace them with their positive opposites. We replace "worthless" with "worthwhile," "unlovable" with "lovable and loving." Old traumas can be healed, and old unwholesome self beliefs can be released.

We used to believe that personality wasn't mutable, that we couldn't change who we had become. That isn't necessarily true. We can leave in place the positive and neutral self concepts and beliefs that make us who we are, but we can actually remove from our subconscious the self concepts that prevent us from being and doing all that we can— physically, emotionally, spiritually, and in our behavior and relationships.

Chapter 4
OUR 10 CORE FEARS, NEGATIVE SELF CONCEPTS AND BELIEFS

Each of us has a unique set of negative self concepts and beliefs. There are some that are so powerful, and so pervasive, that most of us have them to greater or lesser extent. Consciously, we do not generally have even the slightest clue we are acting upon them.

This chapter is about ten of these powerfully negative self concepts and beliefs that I have found are predominant. Generally, they produce fear within an individual, and, cause maladaptive, self defeating conduct. The fear these ten produce may be mild, to quite anxious or raised to the level of panic stricken. In regards to the top ten, the words "fears," "negative self concepts" and "negative beliefs" are virtually interchangeable.

Self concepts are simply beliefs about ourselves. We often develop negative self concepts and beliefs in response to fear—and these negatives are often, themselves, fears that then become self-fulfilling prophecies. In their extreme forms, they can be life-threatening. In their milder forms, they can simply impede the quality of our lives. "I am unlovable," for instance, can result in death by starvation in the form of anorexia. In a less intense version, it might show up as living alone.

The core fears described in this chapter are by no means the only ones. They are simply the ones that I see as so critical. In my experience, most of our physical and psychological problems have their roots in one or more of these core fears, or negative self concepts and beliefs.

Although some fears and negative beliefs are frequently associated with a particular dis-ease, there is no direct correlation. Almost any fear or belief can contribute to any dis-ease—and one negative can branch out into more than one dis-ease. "I deserve to be abandoned," for instance, might be at the core of both depression and smoking let alone Borderline Personality Disorder. Regardless of the issues that clients present, the Core Healing process remains the same. Our job is to find the negatives, delete them, and replace them—and at the same time, and quite opportunistically, reframe historical trauma from the mature perspective of the now.

In the stories that follow, you will see how these fears tend to overlap with one another. You will also see that, as we work with them in the Core Healing process, they lose their power over us. Here are the top ten core fears, in the form of negative self concepts or beliefs:

1. I deserve to be abandoned by others, self and/or God.

About 98% of my clients over the past twenty years have had this core fear—yet very few of them were aware of it when we started working together. "I deserve to be abandoned" is powerful and insidious, in part because it is usually hidden from our conscious awareness.

"I deserve to be abandoned" is almost always present with depression, and I believe that self abandonment is the basis of almost every addiction. The relationship between high divorce rates and this belief about abandonment is obvious. Pick enough fights with your spouse and voila....the spouse gets fed up and leaves you. Other consequences may be rage, isolation, feelings of not being lovable or good enough, social anxiety, poor self care, and extreme fear of being alone. People who come to me for help with significant problems almost always carry this fear.

The fear of abandonment is a fear of being left alone, of not having anyone there for us, and/or of being rejected—physically, emotionally, or spiritually. It generates anger and a host of other related fears. This core fear has a logical progression. If I deserve to be abandoned by others, why shouldn't I abandon myself? Self abandonment, left unchecked, leads to suicide. If I believe in God, there may be the intermediary next step of feeling abandoned by God—or wanting to push God away. If I feel abandoned even by God and there is no intervention, I can feel stark terror, which can also lead to insanity and/or suicide. Suicide is self abandonment to the nth degree.

Because so few people are aware of having this core fear, I treat it a little differently from how I treat other problems that clients present. In order to make sure we cover it in our Core Healing sessions—identify it, delete it and everything in its constellation, and replace it with a positive opposite—I always ask new clients if we can deal with it first. Even if they tell me they don't have any fear of abandonment, or any conscious sense that they deserve to be abandoned, I ask, "Would it be alright if we checked it out, just to make sure?" "I deserve to be abandoned" is the only core fear for which I ask such permission. By dealing with abandonment first, I am also trying to inoculate my clients against future "abandonments" and losses. There will always be times in life when we feel abandoned, for example, when a loved one dies or a dear friend leaves the friendship or moves to another city.

    Aaron came to me because the anxiety attacks that he had experienced since he was a young man had become so severe as he approached forty that he could no longer even go into his office. Aaron had been raised in an observant Jewish home and, with the encouragement of his mother, had even studied to be a rabbi, but had chosen instead a career as a software executive. Through the Core Healing process, he realized that his decision to "abandon" being a rabbi, a position his non-religious father ridiculed, and instead "go for a real man's job," had resulted in a subconscious belief that he had abandoned God—and so he deserved to be abandoned by God. He went back to that decision and his early moments of panic about it. He was guided to relive those events from a new, and kinder, perspective. We dissolved the fear of being abandoned by God, and replaced it with what he knew in his heart to be true: "I love God, and God loves me and cares for me."

    After our work together, Aaron told me, "You know, at first I wondered why I had to suffer so much, why God didn't just take away my anxiety. But then I realized 'God helps those who help themselves.' If He'd done all the work for me, I wouldn't have learned how to deal with this myself. I wouldn't have gotten to that subconscious belief—and others—and I wouldn't be as strong as I am now."

    Different people abandon themselves in different ways. Some of the most common ways we abandon ourselves are smoking, obesity, unhealthy habits, drugs, suicide, not allowing ourselves to succeed, or not allowing ourselves love.

2. I deserve to punish, be punished, and punishment changes bad behavior.

    This is another self concept that is fear-based, and that most of us share. In this context, punishment means brutality toward oneself, inviting brutality from another, or imposing brutality on others.

    Punishment, a disastrous concept, keeps us in whatever is the problem. Out of a fear of punishment, we may alter our behavior, but at what price? The development of additional negative self concepts and beliefs. Karl Menninger wrote a book entitled <u>The Crime of Punishment</u>. I never read the book, but I love the title. My work with hundreds of people so validates that notion.

If we strive for compassion, let alone healing, we cannot, we must not endorse punishment. *Rather than punishment*, I endorse sequestering, community service, remuneration, time out, "no" meaning "no," structure, and for those amenable, Core Healing.

Punishment engenders fear, pain, rebelliousness, anger and rage, all of which foster feelings of being out of control. Feeling out of control fosters anxiety and leads to depression. Depression can lead to despair, the conundrum of feeling trapped or clueless what to do next, which can then lead to suicide.

The most brutal punishment I witness is self punishment. We punish ourselves for many reasons not the least of which is in response to feelings of outrage with ourselves for doing something that we judge to be incredibly "stupid." That subconscious self punishment decision can lead to the ongoing enervation and joylessness of depression at worst or to a milder form of depression that comes from years of "beating oneself up" with nasty self name calling, and, the punitive feeling of guilt.

We have been programmed by society and by many religions that punishment assuages pain, mitigates feelings of helplessness and betrayal, and makes us "good" again. We have been taught that punishment is the only way to make up for some things.

I first worked with Arlene on relationship issues when she was twenty-five. Those issues were resolved, but Arlene returned a year later suffering from depression. We talked about what was going on in her life and she told me, "You know, it's the strangest thing. I'm not dating anymore. The only guys I hang out with are gay. I go to gay bars and dance with them. I know I'm not gay, but I'm hanging out in gay places. What am I doing?"

Under hypnosis, I asked her subconscious mind to return to the most critical, most relevant memory to this issue. She remembered an abortion. I asked her how she felt about it. "Like I'd done something terrible. Like I'd killed somebody," she responded. Her negative self concept was, "I am a killer of babies, and I deserve to be punished." We worked with this negative some more, in ways that will be elaborated upon in Chapter 6. Arlene also realized that she had decided, "I will never fall in love again.," which actualized as an onerous negative reactive decision. The punishment of brutal aloneness from appropriate company in terms of her heterosexual orientation not only fit the "crime" but served prophylactic purpose. Moreover, by never falling in love again, she believed that no mistake could happen again, no fetus aborted. Because Arlene was heterosexual and enjoyed the company of men, her subconscious solution was to hang out with gay men. By seeing only gay guys, she knew she would not fall in love and that therefore getting pregnant would become a non issue. By never becoming pregnant again, she could not commit a terrible act again.

In the healing phase of the Core Healing process, Arlene was reminded that all she need do is ask forgiveness of God and it is forgiven. With obvious repentance in her heart, she did. She was also led to forgive herself and to reject the concept of punishment. Punishment primarily serves enslavement and entrenchment in the problem in need of correction. In addition, Arlene committed to the kind of conduct with the next heterosexual male she fell in love with, the kind of love that came naturally to her, that would not place her in such predicament again. Finally, she was led to experience the Eternal Spirit of her unborn child and know that in God's embrace the Spirit of the child lives on.

I am thrilled to report that Arlene is now married and has two children who she treats with greater appreciation than words can begin to express.

3. I'm not good enough.

This core fear can also take the form of not being smart enough, pretty enough, not managing time well enough, not being important enough, or *anything* enough. It is strongly connected to feelings of being bad, worthless, weak, lazy, irrelevant, inferior, scared, angry, inadequate, unworthy of unconditional love, a failure, a loser, nervous or stressed.

Again, you can see that this core fear overlaps with other fears, self concepts and beliefs. And again, it can move in any direction to create problems, depending on the person's other self concepts and beliefs.

Cory had an IQ of 163, but had difficulty passing tests in college. He had gotten excellent grades in high school, which made his academic trouble even more mystifying. In Core Healing, he got in touch with the source of his difficulty with tests. Cory was the first person in his family ever to attend college, and they made it clear that he was "rising above himself." They loved him and were proud of him, but they also shook their heads in disbelief that someone with his background was doing something that none of them had ever been able to do. Cory arrived on campus subconsciously believing that he didn't belong, and that he wasn't on the same level with the other students despite his obvious intelligence. "I'm not good enough" swung into action. He said he felt like a "bad seed," as if his genetics (which erroneously were believed to be "not good enough") would overcome his talents. His conscious mind did as it was told by his subconscious, and he started failing tests.

Once Cory had identified the source of the problem under hypnosis, we could delete the negative constellation of beliefs associated with "not being good enough" and replace it with one that served him well: "It's okay to succeed in college and in life, and, that regardless of his genetic make-up there is no bad seed gene."

4. I have to be perfect.

This core fear is different from a healthy pursuit of excellence (Gardner, 1961). It is the feeling that we have to do everything just right—and that we are in danger if we fall short of perfection. At its worst, this self concept can result in behavior that is obsessive, compulsive, and/or ritualistic—all of which are mismanagement of the intense anxiety regarding falling short of perfection. Indecisiveness is also a hallmark of this fear, since any decision could result in less than a perfect one.

Like the fear of abandonment, the fear of not being perfect, at its zenith, is primal, a "scared to death" fear. People who suffer from it in the extreme can literally be afraid subconsciously that they will die if they are not perfect. They "reason" that if they are not perfect, they will not be loved. If they are not loved, they will be alone. If they are alone and abandoned, they will die. In childhood, such a sequence would be true. That is where such fears are developed.

Most people with this core fear had parents who wanted to be "perfect parents." If you want to be a perfect parent, you need to have a perfect child. These parents can become extremely controlling, which is stressful to all concerned. Threats of punishment for lack of perfection may be implied or expressed, physical or emotional—but children get the message. Children who are overly controlled generally grow up intimidated into behaving as perfectly as they can. They are coerced into dependency on their parents, which intensifies their need to be perfect.

Jane had wanted to be a doctor from the time she was five years old. Her parents were thrilled, and she did well in college and medical school. But her first rotation as an intern was in the Emergency Room, and during her first week she saw three people die. She quit and went home to live with her dismayed parents. By the time she came to see me, she had become severely depressed.

Consciously, Jane realized she did not have to be perfect. She "just wanted to do a good job," which was a reasonable expectation. But under hypnosis, she became aware of the depth of her drive toward perfection. In the ER, she and the other doctors had not been perfect. People had died. Further, she was now living in the same home where her need to be perfect had been planted and nurtured by her parents. "I have to be perfect" was getting systematically reinforced—and she knew that she was not perfect. Hence, the depression that had brought her to Core Healing.

She relinquished and replaced her need to be perfect with a better constellation. "My best is highly qualified and yes, I may in spite of all medical efforts lose a patient, but I know now I will have done my very best and my best is very good enough to save many lives." "Moreover, I am worthy of respect for my commitment to quality effort because who I am is a woman, a physician, of excellence."

5. I can't and/or don't want to be responsible for myself.

> "One needs a will....(that is) apt always
> to total acceptance of every consequence
> of living and dying."   Morris West

Like "I have to be perfect," this core fear often starts with parents who are overly protective, overly controlling, overly demanding, overly delegating, overly excusing from appropriate consequence to a misbehavior (Dreikurs, 1972), frightfully punitive in orientation or dependent on their children. Ideally, parents teach their children self control—the capacity to act within acceptable boundaries that do not harm themselves or others, and to make their own decisions and set their own limits. But when parents have all the control, children do not learn to be responsible for themselves. They learn to look outside themselves for control, guidance, and boundaries. They are not in charge, they are not responsible for their own lives; others are. That "other" may be whatever authority figure is handy—a boss, a mate, anyone to whom the person can look to see what he or she should be, do, or have—or it may even be a "thing" like food. People who are "out of control" with eating are often looking outside themselves for something to take charge—in this case, food can become a way to take control of feelings, for example. As a result, it becomes an irresponsible choice.

A colleague of mine by the name of Bede Smith, taught me to look at the word responsible in terms of its parts. Respond - able. We need to be equipped with the ability to appropriately respond as opposed to react to any given situation. If we were taught like one of my client's, we would be in great shape. After doing hypnosis with this fellow to quit smoking, it was his conviction that he had not been hypnotized. And, he said so as he dutifully paid his bill. About three hours later, this gentleman, and I use the word gentleman advisedly, called me back. He said, "mam, I just had to call you". "For you see mam, my mama raised me to be the kind of man that if I make a mistake, I am to own up to it". "Well mam, I'm not smoking, I guess I was hypnotized". I love this story and repeat it in the therapeutic setting every chance I get for several edifying reasons. This fellow was taught how to be in constructive, responsible control of his conduct.

Well meaning parents can do too much and make too many excuses for their children. They can rob them of how to take responsibility for their own mistakes. When parents provide an overly protective environment, children simply don't learn how to function in the world. The idea that they might have to go out on their own, be responsible for themselves as unprepared as they know they are can be terrifying.

They simply don't have basic life skills:
- *Practical skills* like balancing a checkbook, choosing an appropriate wardrobe, cooking, holding down a job, time management, and even doing laundry.
- *Relational skills* like negotiation, compromise, anger resolution, working through differences and being able to own up when at fault.
- *Emotional skills* like managing their levels of stress and anger.

When children who have been raised in an overly protective environment get close to an age at which it is no longer appropriate for them to live with their parent, they often panic and do whatever is necessary to avoid being out on their own. This might include not being able or willing to find a job, developing a mental or physical disorder, or creating some situation or condition that makes it "impossible" for them to find their own way in life. This core fear can translate into: "I'm not supposed to be in control of myself; everyone in authority in my life is supposed to be in control" or "I can't make it on my own." So they foster a life of dependence, which in the extreme can lead to being institutionalized. Responsibility for self there is minimal.

I am not supposed to be, am not able to be, I don't know how to be or I refuse to be responsible for myself also shows up when children have been either neglected—and therefore not learned basic life skills—or given *too much* responsibility. They may, for instance, have been put in charge of caring for a younger sibling and received the message that if anything bad happened, they were to blame.

As a child is being raised and being responsible becomes associated with punishment, a fear of mistakes, failure, fault, and consequences will occur to more or less degree depending on how frighteningly the parents come across. Significantly frightened children will become significantly frightened adults who will avoid being responsible at all costs. "Pass the buck," becomes their norm.

Another variation on this theme of fearing or even resenting responsibility occurs when parents make their children feel responsible for them and their happiness. Ray had an alcoholic mother who expected him to clean up after her, fix dinner, and have the house in order by the time his father got home from work. He ran from any such responsibilities as an adult, and refused to share household duties with his spouse. He developed a fear of overload or pressure, a deep resentment, and a feeling of being out of control that led to depression. Moreover, it is not surprising that his marital relationship suffered as well.

This core fear can also manifest as its opposite: "I have to be responsible for everyone and everything." These people take on responsibilities that are not theirs to take—for the happiness of other people in their lives, inappropriate financial responsibilities, doing others' work, etc. They were raised to believe that this is what they are supposed to do. These people need to differentiate between appropriate and inappropriate arenas in which to take responsibility, and give other people the opportunity to be responsible for *them*selves.

6. I'm out of control.

This core fear manifests as an almost dizzying sense of not knowing what to do, or where to turn. It can be about family, raising a child, a job, a relationship, an emotion such as anxiety, or life in general. Feeling significantly out of control is often the step just before a person sinks into deep depression, so it is important to get help when this fear arises.

Many people who have the self concept, "I am not the one who is supposed to control my life," *depend* on others. They may also turn to a substance to *depend* upon for controlling how they feel. The irony here is that this approach to self management that is outside oneself leads to feeling even more out of control. Feeling out of control or other-controlled leads to anxiety and depression. At its worst, feeling supremely out of control makes a person feel so scared they feel as if they are going crazy. They can feel like they are headed into a terrifying unknown that heightens their panic. When feeling chronically terrified and helpless, insanity can become a release into total dependency.

One clue that this fear is starting to take over is the phrase, "I can't handle it anymore." When you hear these words, or when you think or say them, know that it is time to get immediate help. Often what people mean by these words is, "I need to take a mental vacation, to be taken care of by someone else." They may be about to abandon responsibility for themselves.

There is a very wide gradient here, and it is important to see where the person is along that gradient. It can mean anything from "I need a break. I think I'll spend a week at a spa," to staying with a friend in a distant city, to entering a psychiatric institution, to committing suicide.

Jennifer had quit her job and gone out on her own as a graphic artist. She thought it would be great to be her own boss and set her own hours, but after a year, she was beside herself. The organizational skills that had made her such a star at her old firm seemed to evaporate, and she felt like she was going in a million directions at once—marketing, meeting with prospects, keeping up her portfolio, not to mention the actual work of doing designs for clients. Her situation was, by its nature, somewhat stressful—but Jennifer was normally on top of things, and her feeling of being out of control now was so acute that some days, she couldn't even get out of bed.

Under hypnosis, she returned to a time when she was three. She was playing in her room and had all her toys and dolls out. Her mother came into the room and screamed, "What's the matter with you? You're totally out of control!" She began slamming toys into Jennifer's toy box while saying, "A place for everything, and everything in its place." Jennifer was unwittingly traumatized by her mother. So what the mother said, how Jennifer felt, the frightening memory itself was imprinted upon Jennifer's subconscious awaiting an 'appropriate' time to come into play.

Jennifer's core fear was that in her own room, her own space, she was out of control. And one thing was clear: In her home office, there was not a place for everything and everything was not in its place. At the firm, working within the company's systems and its organizational structure had kept her "in line," as she said. But now, on her own, in her space and not theirs, this core fear raised its head.

After we deleted and replaced Jennifer's negative constellation with a positive one, including making her aware that she could replicate the organizational structure of the work environment when she was an employee into the self employed environment of her home, she could now work without undue stress or anxiety. She was able to roll with the punches, and to enjoy her creative work. She had the Core Healing bonus of an internal resolution with her mother's mismanagement of her as a child.

7. I am unlovable.

Most of us have this core fear as well. As children, we all wanted to be loved just as we were, without conditions. Very few of us were loved this way, or as much as we wanted to be—or as much as we deserved. We often think of ourselves as unlovable as we are. This sense of not being lovable enough as we are can become part and parcel of an eating disorder which is discussed in more detail in Chapter 11.

We often associate the fear of not being lovable in the context of relationships, but it can go in almost any direction and be at the root of any of the dis-eases in Part 2 of this book.

Janet was three when her little brother was born. Until then, she had been her mother and father's little girl, their only child and the focus of their lives. With the new baby's arrival, all the attention went to him. This was both exciting and horrible for Janet. She had a new brother, people came to visit, and there was a lot of activity in the house. But then, the baby didn't go back to the hospital. Janet never regained her parents' attention at the level it had been. Although her parents bent over backward to make her feel special, it was never really the same.

Not much changed on the outside. She was still well behaved, with only the normal amount of sibling rivalry. She did well in school, although her father realized that she wasn't working up to her potential. She had boyfriends as a teenager, but the relationships never lasted long. She was married and divorced twice by the time she was thirty.

The crisis came when Janet was thirty-two. She had worked for a particular company for eight years and given her heart and soul to it. But there was bitter internal strife in the workplace, and Janet found herself not only passed over for a promotion, but ousted from the entire organization. She was crushed—and furious. She started overeating and within three months had gained twenty pounds. This result was about punishment and mismanagement of emotions. Then, on top of all that, she beat herself up with harsh negative self talk mercilessly.

When Janet came to see me, we talked about her anger over being fired. Under hypnosis, her most critical, most relevant memory was a day soon after her little brother came home from the hospital. Janet had wanted her mother to help her get dressed and the mother shouted over her shoulder, "Leave me alone, Janet, can't you see I'm busy with the baby?" This was an unusually brusque response from Janet's mother, who that day was simply at the end of her rope with two young children. But in Janet's state of stress and fear, the self concept that got imprinted on her subconscious was, "I am unlovable, and unworthy of helpful attention." That self concept had been lurking in her subconscious for decades, especially in her relationships. It took trouble at work, where Janet placed most of her self esteem and value, to prompt her to seek help.

At work, it was a sink or swim environment. No attention, no help was given those drowning. No care given. Just savage dismissal. When she could see the similarity as to what was actually instigating her problems, Janet was in a position to delete that self concept and replace it with "I deserve to be loved unconditionally, and most especially by me." Janet was also programmed to realize that while she deserved to be loved and to be loved unconditionally, that so long as she treats others respectfully, not to take it personally if someone doesn't appreciate let alone love her. Not everyone a person meets can be expected to have that depth of reaction.

Janet was aided in forgiving herself and not treat herself harshly as she felt her mother had that day. Losing weight was an appropriate consequence to loving oneself unconditionally.

8. I'm afraid to be alone.

This core fear usually gets imprinted very early in life. For infants and young children, being alone can trigger a fear of death. They are helpless and powerless, and these are the feelings that often accompany "I'm afraid to be alone" into adulthood. Because of its potential connection to the fear of death, this fear also bleeds into the fear of the unknown—or what might happen after death.

Jim's physical experience was like that of most babies born in hospitals before the need for immediate bonding with the mother was understood. He was taken from his mother and placed in an infant basket in the nursery while his mother slept and rested. But subconsciously, his reaction was "I am alone, and therefore I'm going to die." As he grew up, whenever his parents left the room, he became distraught. At school, he always moved in a large crowd of guys. When he got old enough to date, he was never without a girlfriend.

Jim came to me because he had been convicted on a domestic violence charge. He said he no longer loved his wife Karen, but he couldn't leave her. The situation enraged him, and he had beaten her up twice subconsciously trying to get her to abandon him. He was in tears as he told me this, and I saw that he truly wanted to put this issue to rest.

In the Core Healing process, through hypnotic age regression, Jim relived that time in the infant basket in the hospital. He experienced the emotions, became clear on the source of the self concept that he could not be alone, and in the healing phase we replaced it with "I am capable and lovable, and can take care of myself on my own as well as share my life with others." Six months later, he and Karen got an amiable divorce. He waited a year before he married a woman with whom he has two children and a loving family. He says he is never tempted to violence, not only because of our work on that issue but also because he doesn't feel trapped anymore. He is grateful for every day of this new life.

9. I'm stupid.

Most of us are afraid of looking, sounding, or acting stupid—or of appearing inferior in any way. We are *terrified* of the humiliation associated with a gaff. As children, "dumb mistakes" generally led to ridicule.

"Stupid" means different things to different people. It might be a question of intellect, or of making "stupid" mistakes in life, or not being street smart as in being savvy, or being "dumb" about relationships, or anything we believe is "stupid." Most of us avoid people and situations that provoke the least fear of looking stupid, and are inclined to beat ourselves up if we catch ourselves doing something we consider "stupid"—even when others don't notice it. Fears of failure, humiliation, or ridicule as mentioned earlier are ancillary to this core fear.

Mary did well in college and law school, but instead of taking the bar exam she decided to work as a paralegal for awhile, "just to get an idea of how various firms work, and where I want to wind up." Two years passed, and she still hadn't taken the bar. Since she was so bright, the partners at the firms where she worked could never understand why she didn't take the exam, and urged her to do so. Mary became less and less willing to endure the stress that surrounded taking the bar. Over time, her fear became overwhelming.

When we started working together, she had bitten her nails down to stumps and appeared nervous and agitated. She had begun to have panic attacks at work that were affecting her performance. When I asked her, under hypnosis, about the most critical, most relevant memory to her fear of taking the bar, she saw herself at the dinner table, the night before the SAT's. Her father was lecturing her on how important the test was, because it would determine the college where she was admitted. "You'd better do well, honey," he said, "because your mother and I have sacrificed a lot to send you to a good school and it would be a shame if you came across as too stupid to get in."

In her panic, Mary had internalized the idea that her father thought she might be stupid. She idolized him. If that's what he thought of her, it must be true. The idea had stuck with her the next day. Despite being very intelligent and having gotten excellent grades in high school, Mary didn't do as well as expected on the SAT's. And she did not, in fact, get into the university where her parents had hoped to send her. "I'm stupid" was now firmly in place. Taking the bar exam was yet another big test, another opportunity to appear stupid—and her subconscious simply would not let her near it! Once Mary realized what she was actually doing and we had dissolved all the negatives surrounding and including "I'm stupid" and replaced them with "I am an intelligent, competent woman," her anxiety dissolved as well. She signed up for the bar, and took and passed it six months later.

10. I can't take the pain.

We all experience pain, but we work through it and life returns to normal. When the belief that we *can't take* the pain gets imprinted on our subconscious, it becomes destructive. Pain becomes something to be avoided at all costs because, "Next time, I don't think I can pull myself out."

This "never again" reaction can result in behaviors that range from weight gain, to refusal to remarry, to never getting involved in relationships or even friendships, to actions that become increasingly self destructive.

Wendy married young and immediately had two little girls. A year later, her husband left her and disappeared. She had no job, and no child support. Fortunately, her mother lived nearby and could take the children while Wendy worked double shifts as a checker at a large supermarket. She made good money, spent it wisely, gave her kids everything they needed, and eventually was able to pay for child care when they were not in school and free up her mother's time.

On the outside, Wendy looked like she was coping well—but she started feeling increasingly sad and depressed. She never dated, refused to be fixed up by her co-workers, and didn't even go out with friends. She told me, "I don't have time, and just don't see the point. I'm exhausted when I get home. All I want to do is have a drink and stare at TV until I can get to sleep, so I can get up and do the same thing the next day. I think I was running on adrenalin when the kids were young. Now that they're in school and I have some breathing room, I find myself becoming more and more depressed. But I'm sure not gonna have another relationship. I know where that leads, and I couldn't take it again!"

Under hypnosis, Wendy saw that, in the fear and panic right after her husband left, a thought she had became imprinted on her subconscious, "I can't take the pain. To avoid such pain happening again, I will never have another relationship." She had put herself on automatic, done what needed to be done for the girls, and never looked back. But now the pain of her isolation was as great as the pain of her husband leaving. She was willing to let go of "I can't take the pain" and replace that negative self concept with "I am open to what life brings, move through pain when it happens and move on, willing to love again." Wendy's children were flower girls at her wedding two years later.

DEALING WITH CORE FEARS

These are among the key fears some or all of which may become lodged in the subconscious as negative self concepts and beliefs. They bleed and blend into one another, as well as into other fears. Each has its own particular set of constellations. It is crucial to assume the potential of their presence and to weed out these fears as negative self concepts and beliefs. Unchallenged, they breed anxiety, anger, and depression—and lead inevitably to the types of dis-eases of Part 2.

We can help our children eradicate or at least minimize these fears by teaching them that caution may be useful, but that extreme fears are unnecessary if we are prepared for life's challenges. For instance, martial arts training can mitigate the natural fear they may feel on the streets. Children need to know that there is danger in the world, that it is wise to be somewhat wary, but that fear is unnecessary and that skills can be learned, and precautions can be taken to ensure appropriate responses to the dangers inherent in life.

In this chapter, we have talked about people who identified, dissolved, and replaced their subconscious negative self concepts and beliefs. In the next two chapters, we will elaborate on how that is done.

Chapter 5
CORE HEALING:
What It Does

We have seen that the subconscious mind governs our behavior, our relationships, our emotions, and even our bodies. When positive beliefs are activated, life goes well. When negative beliefs are activated, we experience pain, distress, and dis-ease—regardless of what we want, strive for, or think possible with our conscious minds.

Clearly, the way to a more joyful, productive life is to bring to conscious awareness one's negative self concepts and beliefs, dissolve them and replace these negatives with their positive opposites. This marvelous adventure requires avoiding the temptation of denial as to the source beliefs and fears. One must rather embrace the golden unknown, the truth of one's own perceptions, and, surface this knowledge that opens the door to transcendence. This is the purpose and the result of Core Healing.

It is no small bonus that with a Core Healing commitment much is derived such as: past trauma are desensitized and reframed to positive purpose; an assertive adult stance becomes the norm; the mantle of responsibility is assumed, and, imprinted is how to use responsibility to mitigate inappropriate anger. Moreover, there is the implantation of the values facilitative of fearless, secure and compassionate living. The less fear in which a person comports themselves the more confidently they stride through life. The less the fear, the less the anger. The less the anger, the less the depression. The less the depression, the more energy for love. The more energy for love, the more joy and serenity.

WE DO, AND WE DO NOT, HAVE CHOICES

The premise of Core Healing is the liberation of self for the purpose of being able to make a broad range of loving and wise choices. The freedom to choose is not the given generally ascribed to the circumstance of being human. *Our subconscious programming <u>dictates</u> our choices. Our subconscious governs our emotions, our behavior, our relationships, our health and the quality of our Spiritual life.* If we want the glory of the right to make our own true choices, our subconscious must have been educated during our developmental years to facilitate independent, self controlled, autonomous, responsible and loving conduct. Otherwise, we can become the victim of the negative self concepts and beliefs of others. Using one's body to detonate an explosive device is such a case in point.

Personality is a way of describing in generalizations, the effects of the accumulation of all the positive and negative self concepts and beliefs of an individual. In clinical psychological terms, the negative aspects of personality have been described with labels such as depressed, histrionic, bi-polar, anxiety disordered, antisocial, etc. With Core Healing, we now know how relatively swiftly the negative aspects of personality are mutable. Negative aspects of one's own personality can be redesigned to suit the wishes of the client. With access to the subconscious, we can discover the actual, problematic self concepts and beliefs. It is the truth of the client's constellations of negatives that we seek not those of the therapist's or anyone else's. Uncovered, those negatives can easily be deleted and replaced with positive opposites. Problems then simply dissolve. They evaporate, almost as if they never existed. Wise choices which could not be actualized before are now free to be acted upon. The negatives are not there to block their implementation.

With Core Healing, we have a wealth of technology available with which to reconstruct aspects of ourselves that are painful or outdated, destructive or unhealthy, and to get the help necessary to rebuild ourselves in ways that bring peace, joy, and fulfillment to ourselves, to others, and to the world.

Core Healing isn't for everyone. People who succeed with Core Healing are those who are willing to look under the hood, tell the truth about what they see, and have faith that the new parts will work. Excluded from the Core Healing process are those who have a plethora of terrifying childhood experiences, or multiple personalities.

THE GOALS OF CORE HEALING

Core Healing aims to retrieve our birthright to be happy and use ourselves to maximize our full potential, so that we can live in freedom, autonomy, dignity, and happiness. Plain and simple, in doing this our choices become more wise.

Core Healing does not depend upon the therapist using lists of negative beliefs to determine what fears, negative self concepts and beliefs are causing trouble. This process is client centered (Rogers, 1961) because the perceived truth is in the client not in the therapist. The subconscious of the client is explored to unearth these perceived truths. Core Healing employs various hypnoanalytic methods. One is Ideomotor Signaling (Cheek, 1994 and Ewin, 2006). Another is hypnotic age regression (Hammond, 1990). As people get in touch with earlier traumas and their various effects through regression hypnosis, the negative effects can be processed into a healthy adult perspective. We reframe the memories so that they nourish the person's sense of self, and plant the seeds of new, positive outlooks and beliefs. We are literally, linguistically, rewiring the brain by replacing old reactive decisions with positive self concepts and beliefs and by overwriting ugly history with optimistic vistas so that the person is no longer held back from full expression, forgiveness, love of self and others, serenity, or success.

Among the specific goals of Core Healing are:

- Healing old traumas—for the hurt child (Riese, 1966), teen, and adult
- Identifying, deleting, and replacing the negative self concepts and beliefs behind the client's presenting dis-eases
- If there is one, getting to an "Aha!" experience, the one behind a problem at the subconscious level, which facilitates immediate and permanent release
- Removing negative emotions, desensitizing negative memories, and healing hurtful relationships, including the client's relationship with God
- Creating templates at the subconscious level for assertive, adult-to-adult relationships
- Releasing anger and hatred, and stepping into a life characterized by peace, forgiveness, love, and the capacity to live and let live without fear or domination
- Being responsible for our lives and learning from mistakes with dignity, without shame or blame
- Learning to resolve conflicts based on respect and appreciation, rather than on the unfortunate models inherent in past traumas thus alleviating the need to protect and control
- Maximizing our potential through self awareness, self appreciation and embracing life as sacred

- Actualizing our dreams, and fulfilling a sense of purpose with our lives - each of us based on our unique talents and abilities
- Transmitting the above gifts to our children and moving the world toward peace, one person at a time

When such goals are achieved, then we are more likely, *more readily able* to *consistently* attract bounteousness into our lives and those of others. (Byrne, 2006)

FORGIVENESS

Forgiveness is an essential part of Core Healing. We have seen that forgiving someone or self doesn't mean that you condone what they or you yourself did. It simply means that you are willing to let go of the pain and anger surrounding the event, and to stop blaming them or stewing in anger with yourself. You aren't saying that what they did or what you did was okay, or even that you necessarily want them in your life. You are simply saying that you are willing to let go of the pain and anger, so that it won't lodge in your body harmfully, affect your emotions negatively, or decay your spirit.

Without forgiveness, healing cannot take place. If we hold on to the pain and anger, we limit our capacity for changing negative beliefs or replacing them with positive opposites. Before I begin Core Healing with new clients, I always ask them if they are willing to commit to being forgiving. And I explain why. Old traumas may involve perpetrators—caretakers, parents, teachers, coaches, strangers, anyone who has inflicted physical or emotional pain—and these relationships need to be dealt with in a forgiving way. Without my clients' agreement to partner in forgiveness, there is no point in going forward. Without forgiveness, the pain and destruction of these traumas carry on their dirty work.

HOW IT WORKS: Susie's panic attacks

Let's look at one client's experience to get an overview of how Core Healing works before we discuss the specifics.

Susie came to me because she had nearly passed out from a panic attack at the first staff meeting she was to conduct. She was thrilled with her promotion to manager, but had been dreading the staff meeting for a week because she knew she would have to stand up in front of the group. She had rationalized that "hardly anybody likes performing in front of a group, and I'm just one of them." But as the day of the staff meeting approached, Susie actually had physical symptoms erupt indicating the inception of a panic reaction—sweaty palms, increased heart rate, and hyperventilation. Tending toward "stinkin' thinkin," no amount of self talk using her conscious mind could ease this anxiety.

Susie's subconscious was already putting out an "appropriate" response to the "danger" of the meeting that would put her in front of a group. And sure enough, she almost did pass out standing in front of the group, and had to cut the meeting short.

As Susie described the situation to me, it became clear that her conscious mind had tried to push these feelings aside and not feel them. She tried telling herself just to do her job. But at the same time, negative self concepts and beliefs were being culled from the archives, and producing a "flight/ fight" reaction. Her conscious mind could not make sense of the high anxiety. As she actually stepped to the front of the room and "soldiered on," her subconscious put out more "flight/ fight" hormones—which created the chemically induced physical turmoil called a panic attack. Susie was now enduring what felt like life threatening, out of control physical feelings that were overwhelming her with fear bordering on terror.

There was a classic intra-psychic battle being waged between Susie's two minds. The more her logical conscious mind fought the urge to run and her computer center the subconscious, urged her to flee (based on earlier trauma history), the more out of control she felt. The subconscious was in charge.

What was it in Susie's subconscious that drove her to feel compelled to run (Ellis, 1975)? Under hypnosis, I asked her subconscious to take us back to the most critical, most relevant memory to the question: "Why did I get a panic attack at the staff meeting?"

The memory that emerged was from second grade. Susie's teacher had called her to the blackboard at the front of the classroom to solve a math problem. She made a mistake. The teacher said, "Sit down, stupid!" The whole class laughed at Susie. In that moment of trauma, the window to her subconscious flew open. With lightening speed, Susie's subconscious imprinted a host of negative self concepts and beliefs. Among them were:

"Performing in front of the room is dangerous."

"I can't trust myself not to make a mistake in front of others."

"I must deserve to be embarrassed and humiliated when performing in front of a group."

"I never want to be in a situation like this again."

"I perform stupidly in front of others."

"I hate working in front of a group because you never know if you're going to be ridiculed."

(Susie might just as easily have made some positive reactive decisions—if the self concepts and beliefs already in place had been different, or if her teacher had handled the situation with more understanding and compassion. She might have decided, for instance, "Mom is good at the times tables. I'll get her to drill me so, next time, I'll be ready." This decision would foster the self concept: "I am a person who does her homework.")

Now it was clear what had happened. The stimulus had been the staff meeting. Susie's subconscious did its job and responded with the "proper" protection, based on its files of negative self concepts and beliefs. Performing in front of a group is "dangerous" even to the extent of feeling scared to death to do so. The appropriate reaction, therefore, was "flight," and a panic attack with all the physical symptoms ensued.

Healing Susie's problem meant not only finding the second grade memory and changing the negative self concepts into positive, but also desensitizing the traumatic memory. While she was in hypnosis and we had access to the subconscious, I guided Susie through an assertive, adult-to-adult confrontation with her second grade teacher (Berne, 1964). This imprinted the constructive discharge of her anger. I call it constructive because Susie's conversation with her teacher was without hostility or expletives. She told the teacher, as a mature adult, the hurtful consequences of her interaction with her child self that day. In the course of this conversation, with the perspective of years, she could place the fault where it belonged. She could forgive the teacher for ridiculing her, even as egregiously bad as the teacher's behavior was, and forgive herself for making the math mistake. An old, consciously forgotten wound was healed, once and for all. This was essentially Inner Child work (Bradshaw, 1990), but done at the level of the subconscious where it actually facilitated changing the negative self concepts formulated by her seven year old self, while at the same time imprinting a healed wound with the adult self now constructively, compassionately in charge.

We also conducted a rehearsal staff meeting under hypnosis (Erikson, 1985). I guided Susie through watching herself successfully conduct the next meeting. She heard 'her' assertive words. They became integrated as positive self concepts regarding being savvy in what to say. Moreover, observing herself as a competent leader, and seeing herself achieving successful conclusion to the staff meeting, all were imprinted for her to draw upon later. Through this rehearsal, where she had conducted a successful staff meeting, her self concept was now I am someone who is adept at conducting staff meetings, and, as a result was ready and even eager to perform!

WHAT MAKES CORE HEALING DIFFERENT?

As I have said, there is no element of Core Healing that is not widely known and used. I think my colleague who was healed of his anxiety disorder put it best: "It's *the way those known elements are put together* that's so unique!"

Core Healing integrates many hypnoanalytic and psychotherapeutic methods into a synergistic whole, bringing to bear the strengths of various techniques to create something that works in deep and potent ways. These are some differences I have noticed, as well as people have pointed out to me, between Core Healing and other therapies:

1. *Core Healing works with each person's subconscious to elicit the actual traumas and truths relevant to the sources of the problem, rather than working from diagnostic descriptions and surmising which diagnosis fits and therefore what course of action is appropriate. Likely, that course of action would include the cognitions in need of reframing.* Most traditionally trained therapists keep the DSM IV (1994) handy. It is an excellent reference for descriptors pertinent to problematic human conditions. Many are astute at seeing what is going on with clients and develop a course of action according to the relevant diagnosis. Cognitive Behavioral therapists have available lists of negative self concepts to select from among them those they deem in need of change. Bottom line, however, this is essentially educated, and yes experienced guessing that relies heavily on the skill and intuition of the therapist.

Core Healing leaves nothing to chance, guesswork, or the acuity of the individual therapist. It does not presume to know the truth about why any particular client is depressed, anxious, or has an eating disorder. Some of the reasons may be quite unique to that individual. Unless we can go directly to the subconscious, where the negative self concepts and beliefs reside, it is difficult to know the whole truth about what is going on. Core Healing literally asks the client's subconscious exactly where the problem originated (the traumatic memory), as well as zooms in on the negative self concepts and beliefs that were absorbed and that are creating the current problem. Knowledge is power. With correct information about the problematic issue, healing becomes easy.

2. *Core Healing goes beyond the presenting problem.* In the medical model, on which we in the field of psychology often base our treatment, a person comes in with an injury such as a fractured leg. X-rays are taken. A medical history is taken. Then the leg is set and placed in a cast. Then there are check up visits. Repair is done. End of story. In the same way, with a client grieving a failed relationship, the therapist might conduct an intake interview, examine the client's history, contract for treatment, explain the plan for resolution, and execute it over several visits. The therapist's plan may be to talk with the client about the importance of dealing with each stage of a grief reaction. As they do so, the therapist will likely suggest some cognitive changes. These shifts, if they occur, will probably reduce the grief reaction. The client feels better, and says, "Thank you." The therapist says, "My pleasure." The client leaves satisfied. The symptoms have been treated, but an opportunity has been missed.

The grief, the pain has subsided. That is certainly good. But a grand opportunity was missed. What negative self concepts and beliefs might the client unwittingly have made while in the throes of the trauma of breaking up? What were the negative self concepts and beliefs that contributed to the break-up? Did the client choose a life's partner wisely? If not why not? And, shouldn't the negatives contributive to fruitless attraction be dealt with?

Core Healing goes beyond what might be considered adequate expectation and in a way that can allow for profound, productive change. We would work not only with the primary beliefs related to the grief, anger, and failed relationship (and with the constellations surrounding them)—but also with all the issues and difficulties the client could identify in his or her life at that time. This thorough approach I call "cleaning house." We would probe the subconscious to reveal as many as 200-400 negative self concepts and beliefs in order to "clean house." In traditional "talk therapy," not the client, or the therapist, neither could possibly guess at the multitude of what the relevant, self defeating beliefs were. Through what I call band-aid hypnotherapy, at best, some may be surfaced and/or intuited. Helpful? "Yes." Thorough? "Doubtful." One issue surfaces at best one full constellation of negatives. Many related yet separate issues will surface many constellations. The more negatives cleared out, the less that is left to haunt the client. The less negatives, the less stressed and the more calm the client feels.

My mantra is: Seek the truth, the whole truth, and nothing but the truth. That is what sets us free. Granted, it is the client's perception of truth, but it is upon their perceptions that their self concepts are formulated.

3. *Core Healing not only heals the particular presenting issue, but inoculates clients against being affected by those same negative self concepts and beliefs in the future.* For instance, the client with the failed relationship might be happy to get some coping mechanisms for dealing with the grief and anger from a traditional therapist—but there would be no guarantee the client wouldn't recreate exactly the same situation with another lover. People often end one relationship (or have it ended for them), only to wind up with the same type of person the next time around.

Because Core Healing deletes the negative self concepts or beliefs that got a person into a failed relationship in the first place, those negatives do not rise up again and recreate the same situation. They are gone, and have been replaced with beliefs that draw the individual to the type of relationship preferred. The "siren call" for getting into another similar and unhealthy relationship is gone. Without the old self concepts lurking around the subconscious, the new and healthier relationship can come in. In these cases, I always ask the client to state clearly the traits he or she would like to be attracted to in the next relationship. I want to facilitate healthy, sustainable attraction.

Included in this package of Core Healing therapy, constructive pain management systems are included. The pain of a deeply felt but lost relationship can feel excruciating and lead to a regrettable negative reactive decision like "I'll never fall in love again" in order to avert such debilitating pain happening again.

4. *Core Healing works at the subconscious level, which is in charge.* Most of the above work is done while the client is under hypnosis, so we are dealing with the problem in the subconscious, where our programming resides. Talk therapies that deal only with the conscious mind are useful for some situations, but hidden

or intractable issues must be dealt with at the level of the subconscious. Cognitive or talk therapy can help people reframe their thinking, facilitate some improvement but real and profound change much more readily occurs at the subconscious level. Using hypnosis removes the hit or miss potential of therapy that only engages the conscious mind therapeutically.

5. *Core Healing surfaces, erases and replaces.* Typical talk therapy primarily erases and replaces that which is consciously available and in need of correction for therapeutic outcome.

THE RESULTS

Based on my clients' anecdotal reports of success, and also on measurements pre- and post-Core Healing on the Minnesota Multiphasic Personality Inventory 2, it seems that we can change personality in constructive ways.

The results that clients report include:
- Healing old wounds
- Achieving constructive control over their minds and behaviors
- Being empowered to implement positive thinking
- Coming to terms with the significant relationships in their lives
- Peace within themselves
- Being less, if at all, fearful
- Heightened self-confidence
- Letting go of self-defeating ways of thinking and behaving
- Feeling centered
- Better relationships with family members
- Being able to attract their heart's desires in their life

Core Healing facilitates peace within each individual soul, so that we now have the potential to become a world of peaceful people. If we but choose to process our anger and fear better and faster within ourselves, there is a better chance for world peace. We can avoid the pitfall of repeating the negative thinking that results in destructive behavior generation after generation, and instead live in the compassion that brings joy to everyone.

These are the aims of Core Healing. In the next chapter, we will look at the specific steps that go into accomplishing these results.

CHAPTER 6
THE CORE HEALING PROCESS:
How It Works

How exactly is Core Healing accomplished? What does it look like? In this chapter, we will explore aspects of the Core Healing process. There are three fundamental parts: Preparation, Discovery, and Healing. Each of these larger parts has several components.

Every client is unique, and we don't use every component mentioned in this chapter with every client. This is simply a treasure chest of tools that can be used as, and if, they are appropriate.

PREPARATION

I spend quite a bit of time preparing clients for the Core Healing process. I want them to be very clear about what we are doing, and to realize that they need to team with me in order to get the best results. I also want to engage their conscious mind as a partner in what we will be doing at the subconscious level, so that its resistance, if any, is minimal.

First, we talk about what they want to accomplish with Core Healing. We discuss what they have tried in the past to heal those particular issues, and what has happened as a result. I explain the differences between Core Healing and what they have tried before, and talk about the principles you have read about in Chapters 1-5.

The Basics

We begin with the basics:
1. The subconscious mind can overrule what we want with our conscious, evaluative mind—and one of Core Healing's jobs is to bring the conscious and subconscious minds into beneficial harmony.
2. Dis-ease, both mental and physical, is caused primarily by subconsciously executed negative self concepts and beliefs, learned unhealthy physical habits, and the learned, and predominantly fruitless and exhausting bad habit of worry. Moreover, in order to worry well, the individual must be

steeped in negative thought processes including but by no means limited to thinking and imaging the worst.

3. We can liberate ourselves to actualize wise choices. The subconscious can be accessed in order to discover, delete, and replace negative constellations as well as core heal the all of the individual.
4. Core healing emphasizes a during and post therapy commitment to a form of mindfulness. People must actively assert every effort to create a new habit one that averts stinkin' thinkin'. Skills with which to do that are taught.

If clients resonate with these principles, believe that they will work, and understand that they will be active participants in the process—then we can go forward. People who come to me as referrals or through my website are often on board already. If what I say makes sense to them, if they are committed to a new way of healing, and if they have the expectation that they will heal, then we are off to a good start. They own the process and they are very likely to succeed. If they say or think, "This won't work. Nothing has, and this won't either," then we probably don't have a good match.

It is crucial to enroll the conscious mind in the benefits of Core Healing so that it can support the process. Engaging the conscious mind also makes for harmonious integration and understanding of what has happened—which is useful to charting their future. We also use the conscious mind when learning how to manage feelings and other issues that emerge or re-emerge after our initial sessions together. The culprit is "stinkin' thinkin'." If left unchecked, "stinkin' thinkin'" can cause reinfection. "Stinkin' thinkin'" produces fear and therefore access to the subconscious mind.

Preparation for Hypnosis

I make sure clients understand and are comfortable with the idea of hypnosis, and show them how to use it to their best advantage. I explain that hypnosis opens the door to their subconscious mind, and can give us information about their self concepts and beliefs that the conscious mind cannot. In addition, we can make positive suggestions under hypnosis that the subconscious mind can adopt immediately and completely because we will have deleted the negatives that otherwise would block implementation. Hypnosis is not the healer itself; it simply takes us where we need to go in order to affect the healing. All of this gives us the best possible chance for success.

I let new clients know that I induce hypnosis with progressive relaxation. I simply take them through each part of the body and ask them to relax their feet, legs, abdomen, torso, arms, head, etc. I tell them that anything they feel in hypnosis is fine, and that I will show them how to use whatever they are feeling to their advantage—so that they can bring to our session whatever they are feeling that particular day without any concerns. Feelings can serve as a bridge that takes you where you need to go (Bandler & Grinder, 1981).

I also tell clients about the various levels of hypnosis, and let them know that they may drift among the various levels. Wherever they are is fine. I assure them they do not have to worry about whether or not they "feel" hypnotized. Whether or not they "think" they are hypnotized, they will be so long as they cooperate with The Progressive Relaxation form of induction into the state of hypnosis that I purposely use. This belief in the induction will produce the effect. In addition, I instruct the client that while in hypnosis, I will be asking their subconscious mind to take us back to the most critical, the most relevant memory to their particular issues—and that even if no memory comes up, I have other hypnoanalytic techniques available with which to disclose the negative self concepts and beliefs that are generating the particular problem that we are working on.

I show them how to manage distractions while they are in hypnosis, and even conduct a "rehearsal hypnosis" in which, as I have told them I would do, I make suggestions to their subconscious mind that will be facilitative of our work together going well. I tell them if, for any reason, they ever want to stop a session, just to sit up and open their eyes.

The "Why?" Questions

As part of their homework, I ask clients to make a list of "Why?" questions. These questions refer to any and all of their problems. It is an opportunity to investigate any aspect of their lives. I only want the questions, not the answers, because I will use this list to conduct the Discovery Phase of Core Healing under hypnosis. These "Why?" questions usually point to clients' core fears, negative self concepts and beliefs. They might include questions like:

- Why am I depressed?

- Why do I get anxious when someone else drives?
- Why do I always choose people who leave me?
- Why is my eating out of control?
- Why do I have high blood pressure?
- Why do I smoke?
- Why am I always so stressed?
- Why do I drink too much?
- Why do I get angry so easily?
- Why do I feel at the end of my rope?
- Why do I no longer feel close to God?

They can list as many "Why?" questions as they wish. If they find themselves stumped, or running dry, I give them five words to reflect on to get the juices flowing again: "relationship," "spiritual," "physical," "emotional," and "behavioral." As human beings, these are our primary problem areas. These words can be used to create additional ideas for "Why?" questions.

We will get to the bottom of each one. And in the Healing phase, resolve them.

The Prayer

I only delve into the spiritual component of Core Healing if people want to do so. If they are comfortable with the idea, I ask each new client to write a prayer as part of their homework that begins, "Lord, I pray that through my work here, I may..." Some people object to the word "Lord" because to them, it suggests Jesus. They may prefer the phrase "energy of the universe," or God, or some other reference to the Divine.

It is easier to work with people who have some sense of a divine energy or afterlife (Frankl, 1988). The fears of death and the unknown generally are among our core fears. It is difficult to be completely relaxed and at ease with death and the unknown without some sense of an inviting afterlife or some eternally loving relationship with a pervasive, loving creative energy. Nevertheless, Core Healing can succeed even with atheists or agnostics.

Logistics

While each client is unique, nonetheless, there is an average number of sessions it takes to address all the "Why?" questions, unearth the negatives surrounding them and affect Core Healing. The number of what I call in depth sessions is two to three. The whole Core Healing process takes an additional three to five visits. The visits vary in length. The total amount of time spent is about 10.5 - 14 hours of work. Some of these visits are scheduled 2.5 - 4 hours long. The time configurations can vary somewhat depending upon whether or not I am working with a local or out of town client. We are finished when all of a client's "Why?" questions are fully answered and resolved to their satisfaction. On average, people present with about sixty "Why?" questions, some of which are interrelated.

THE DISCOVERY PHASE

The in depth work of Core Healing usually begins on the third visit. After inducing hypnosis, we initiate the Discovery Phase. We begin probing for negative self concepts and beliefs based on the problems revealed in their "Why?" questions, which they were instructed to prioritize.

The goal of the Discovery Phase is to gather as much data as necessary to accomplish a thoroughgoing outcome in the Healing Phase. Negative self concepts and beliefs are identified, unresolved emotions explored, fears are identified, unresolved relationship issues with their primary care givers and significant others are elicited, pessimistic attitudes surfaced, and, traumas in need of desensitization are fleshed out.

The Discovery Phase of the first in depth session is the most comprehensive and the most important. I ask of every client, if we may begin the session with this why question: "Why might I believe I deserve to be abandoned?" Most clients cannot relate to that idea consciously and deny it as a potential problem. I explain my rationale as to its importance and add that if that issue is a non-issue for them, I will then, in a matter of the few moments it took to check it out, move right on to their number one "Why?" question. (I had no idea when I first started using this process that abandonment issues were so prevalent and so profoundly affecting for just about everyone to some degree or another.)

In each in depth session's Discovery Phase about 10-12 "Why?" questions are addressed. We ask the subconscious for the most critical, most relevant memory to each question. The way I usually phrase this questions is: "Allow your subconscious mind to make you aware of the most critical, most relevant memory to..." That way, we deliberately sidestep the conscious mind, and the client is reminded that we are in an entirely different realm. Also, this phrasing accurately suggests that there is nothing for the client to do other than to relax and *allow* his or her subconscious to bring to awareness what was requested.

The client might go directly to a specific memory, or I might need to probe using one of the hypnoanalytic techniques listed below. Occasionally, no particular memory comes up. Having a specific memory associated with the "Why?" question is important and quite helpful yet not essential to a particular problem's resolution. Sometimes there is no traumatic memory relevant. In that case, a person may become verbally reflective. Helpful thoughts, words, images, feelings can surface through a process of free association that can be so easy in the state of hypnosis. It is like the old fashioned coffee pot that would percolate. Speaking appropriately to the subconscious mind will facilitate material necessary to problem resolution to bubble up.

They may even remember an event "inaccurately," and later discover undeniable evidence that the event didn't actually happen the way they remember it. It doesn't matter what actually happened. *What matters is what it was to* them— *what they think happened, how they felt about it, and the negative self concepts or beliefs that got imprinted on their subconscious as a result.* We are not looking for precision of memory; we are looking for the *effect* of the memory. When the trauma is identified and dealt with constructively in the Healing Phase, the result is serenity—whether or not the traumatic event actually happened the way the client remembers it.

When people start uncovering what is in their subconscious and the pieces of the puzzle start coming together, they often have the freeing and uplifting experience of, "Aha! So *that's* why I do what I do!" Getting that original "Aha!" is wonderful, but we always mine for more to get all the other self concepts and beliefs in that particular constellation. There may be later incidents, or subsequent reinforcing events, that strengthened, expanded, or extrapolated that particular self concept or belief. It might work like this: Say the original incident was being left alone in the crib while Mom went to help the neighbor with her emergency, and the self concept was "I deserve to be abandoned." The infant might feel like nobody was there for her. Then Daddy goes off to work and works late every night. That's a subsequent reinforcing event. Then she goes to school and none of the kids will play with her. Another reinforcing event. She goes on her first date, and he never calls her back. Another reinforcing event. (Parkhill, 1995)

As we've seen, the subconscious imprints thousands of negative self concepts and beliefs in reaction to their life's events. "I am unlovable," for example, might have tens of other self concepts in its constellation, among them: "I'm ugly," "I'm not pretty/handsome enough," "I deserve to be ignored," etc. The goal of Core Healing is to get at the *whole* truth. Accomplishing that results in 100% resolution.

How do we get back to those incidents, and those negative self concepts and beliefs? I use a variety of techniques, depending on what seems appropriate at that particular time for that particular person. These techniques include:

Hypnotic age regression

In hypnosis, I ask the person's subconscious to take us back to when they were a certain age, or to the memory that is most critical, most relevant to their presenting issue.

I use this technique in almost every Discovery Phase, but would not use it with people who were frequently, severely traumatized as children over a long period of time. Reliving those memories might do more harm than good, and actually re-traumatize the person. I also might not use it with people who are dissociative.

Ideomotor Signaling

Rather than verbalizing answers, very often I will ask the client's subconscious to signal "Yes" or "No" to specially phrased questions. One finger is designated as the "Yes" finger and one as the "No". It is a way to let your fingers do the talking versus "the walking." The obvious advantage here is that the person can more readily access their subconscious data files because he or she doesn't have to use their conscious mind to facilitate conversation. Moreover, by-passing the conscious mind more actively allows for swifter retrieval of data.

It takes some practice to phrase questions adroitly to get at the root causes of a person's problems. Be that as it may, the goal is to be thorough in the assembling of all the negative self concepts and beliefs that form the constellation creating the particular problem being addressed. The therapist's knowledge of the types of problematic negative self concepts and beliefs that together might form a particular problem's constellation is very important. *The goal remains, however, to find only those beliefs that are that client's truths. Their truth, their whole truth and nothing but their perceived truths are their passage to freedom.*

Stage setting

We use Stage Setting to gather information about the client's parents and other important people in their lives, and about the negative self concepts and beliefs that imprinted when they were young.

I learned from Dr. Donald Tyrell that we tend to seek out significant others who correspond to the beliefs we absorbed as a result of what we observed our parents or care givers actualizing toward ourselves and toward each other. If, as a little girl I felt prized by my dad, and, unconditionally loved by my mom, and they routinely evidenced genuine affection for each other, I would likely gravitate to a wonderful soul mate who offered me those qualities because they are what I believe I deserve from the most important people in my life. My husband would convey a sense of prizing his relationship with me as well as offer unconditional love. In addition, we would likely be affectionate with each other. Conversely, if as a little girl I felt abandoned by dad and loved by my mom only if I did what she said, then the beliefs about self that their treatment conveyed could attract me into a regrettable relationship. And, if in their relationship I witnessed constant bickering, guess what kind of relationship in which I might likely find myself. While thirsting for unconditional love and the man in my life being there for me, the illusion of which may likely have occurred when courting, after marriage the reality of what I in fact attracted into my life would play out with mounting disappointment. Bickering would be the norm. My husband would likely control me with offering crumbs of love when I did as I was told upon the occasions he was around.

Another example, say a woman's father was an alcoholic. Obviously, her conscious mind is not looking for a man who is an alcoholic—but strangely, that's the kind of man to whom she always seems to be attracted. If she grew up in a home where alcoholic behavior defined "man" and "husband," then the chances are good that, without intervention of some kind, her subconscious will pull her toward men with alcoholic behavior even if not a drinking problem per se. The negative belief imprinted on her subconscious may have been: "Men/husbands are addicts." But the men don't necessarily have to be alcoholics. They just have to display alcoholic or other addictive behavior like smoking or gambling. She might just as easily have come away with the subconscious beliefs, "Husbands are irresponsible or violent—or poor fear managers, or dependent." Not knowing those beliefs are there courts disaster.

I search for this dynamic in clients by asking them to visualize themselves as a six year old, looking up first at one parent, and when concluded, then at the other. I ask the six year old, "If you had one wish, and only one wish, that could come true about one way your mother (father, step-parent, etc.) would have been different, what would it be?" The thing we most wish could have been different about that individual, when peeled down, usually points directly to the negative self concepts or beliefs we will be addressing. This exercise elicits the material with which to "fix" relationship issues. For example, suppose I would have wished that my dad had been home more, that I hadn't seen him only on week-ends. I might well have grown up believing, "I don't deserve the kind of man who is there for me." I might marry a workaholic, or an alcoholic, or someone who traveled constantly for work, or someone who did not know how to be emotionally intimate. Whatever kind of man I chose, the one element that would almost certainly be present is "not there" or "not there much." Suppose I would have wished my mother had been more affectionate with me. A likely self concept would be, "I don't deserve to be treated affectionately." So I might find myself attracted to a guy who is not only a workaholic, but not affectionate either! This dynamic can cross genders and roles.

"Peeling down"

"Peeling down" an issue means asking a series of questions that lead people to the heart of the matter. Each question is designed to take the person a little deeper into the issue. "Peeling down" can lead to a primary fear, self concept, or belief that later we can work on. Other times, we come to the end of the peel down process and the client simply realizes that all the energy around that particular issue has been released.

In hypnosis, Carla recalled an incident when she was five. Her father showed her all his old army gear and said, "If you'd been a boy, I would have given all this to you." She felt sad and angry that she had let him down by not being a boy, and adopted the belief, "My father wanted a boy. I'm not good enough."

Children often blame themselves for everything, and Carla was very angry with herself for not being a boy, giving rise to the reinforcing negative belief, "I deserve to be punished" for doing something wrong by being a girl.

Life went on, and Carla rose to a powerful position in a Chicago corporation. She was known as the "tiger lady" for her frequent outbursts of temper and the brusque, apparently uncaring way she treated some of her staff. Although her sales team produced record-breaking results, there were just too many complaints about Carla and she was advised to seek counseling.

After we discovered the incident with her father, the accompanying rage with herself, and Carla's self concept that "I deserve to be punished," we began to "peel down" this issue.

Therapist: What do you do to punish yourself?

Carla: I work hard. I don't have any fun or play. It's all just work.

Therapist: And because you've grown up feeling like you deserve to be punished, is there anything else that you do?

Carla: Well, I hurt people because their rejection of me is painful.

Therapist: What happens then?

Carla: Then they find some way to get back at me.

Therapist: And when they get back at you, what results?

Carla: I don't get their friendship or cooperation.

Therapist: And then what happens?

Carla: I wind up all alone.

Finally, Carla understood what she was doing. To punish herself, she set people up to abandon her. That left her experiencing the pain of feeling unlovable and alone. (Punishment often takes the form of self abandonment as is implied here. Moreover, self abandonment and abandonment by God become logical next steps to the idea "I deserve to be abandoned.")

In addition to dealing with the original trauma in the Healing Phase, her concept that punishment corrects a mistake and that punishment is apt retribution was changed to punishment serves no useful or loving purpose and only keeps one enmeshed in the mistake. Making amends plus asking forgiveness of self and/or the person aggrieved makes better use of energy now and in the future. We also worked directly on the cessation of self flagellation then and forever in the particular way she had chosen. The inherent goal in all this being to create a more compassionate actively responsible individual.

Once Carla understood the dynamic, and was guided in the loving ways of forgiveness thereby letting the negative energy drain off during the Healing Phase, she was back in control of her life. She was no longer driven. Some of her relationships were now salvageable and some were not. Ugly anger is after all destructive. However, that was a consequence she was now free to responsibly accept (Dreikurs, 1972).

Carla was no longer driven by impulses based on subconscious beliefs she didn't even know were there! She went back to Chicago a person who was not only more effective and inspirational to her team, but someone who could enjoy and relax into being herself—without the constant drive of punitiveness.

Sometimes when we "peel down" to the core of an issue, clients suddenly burst out laughing, even under hypnosis, because they see that the negative self concept or belief—however powerful it may have affected their lives up to that point—actually had very little to do with reality.

Della thought she was ugly, a self concept that had gotten imprinted when she was seven. She had dressed herself to go out to dinner with her parents and brother, but when she came downstairs her mother shouted, "You look awful!"

The "peeling down" of "I'm ugly" went like this:

Therapist: If you're ugly, what will happen?
Della: I won't have any boyfriends.
Therapist: And what will it mean if you don't have any boyfriends?
Della: That I'm a weirdo.
Therapist: And what will happen if you're a weirdo?
Della: Nobody will want to have anything to do with me.
Therapist: And if nobody wants to have anything to do with you, what is your fear?
Della: That I'll wind up alone.
Therapist: And then what?
Della: I'll be a bag lady and die in the gutter.

At this point, Della started laughing. She saw several things at once, and the energy just blew off the whole issue. First, she saw that her fear was not so much about being ugly as it was about abandonment. Second, she saw that, in her case and with her substantial 401K, dying in a gutter was extraordinarily unlikely—

however much she had feared it. We simply followed the issue to its logical conclusion, and nothing was logical about it! We had reached the core fear, blown it, and gone beyond it. In the process, the fear of being ugly simply evaporated.

In the Healing Phase, I would ask Della whether she really wanted to keep fearing all the things we'd talked about in the "peeling down." Of course, she did not. We also talked about whether or not she really was the ugliest person on the face of the earth. Of course, she was not. Neither was she the most beautiful. In truth, like most of us, she was somewhere in between, with some qualities like her figure and skin that many women would consider enviable. Live in the truth, not a negative reactive, exaggerated conclusion. If I am not beautiful, therefore, I must be ugly.

Core Fear Eradication

Through "peeling down" or whatever method is most effective with any particular client, Core Healing strives to get back to the core fear, which itself is a negative self concept, or belief—and to eradicate it. This involves becoming fully aware of our core subconscious fears, self concepts or beliefs, as well as their attendant emotions, and allowing ourselves to experience them. It is important to get beneath whatever fear is being presented to the core fear that underlies it. When you "nail" the core fear, there is a release of energy and that basic fear is eradicated or at least positioned to be eradicated.

For instance, Ted came to me with a fear of being alone. The conversation went something like this:

Therapist: So if you were alone, what would be your fear?
Ted: I'd drink too much.
Therapist: And if you drank too much, what is your fear?
Ted: I wouldn't do anything with my life.
Therapist: And if you didn't do anything with your life, what's your fear?
Ted: I'd feel worthless.
Therapist: And if you felt worthless, what's your fear?
Ted: That I'd kill myself.
Therapist: And if you killed yourself, what's your fear?
Ted: I would go to hell, because I would deserve to be punished by God.

Now we are touching the core fear. Being punished by God was Ted's bottom-line fear. This was not a realization that produced laughter, as Della's had. But it was his truth, his unfortunate conviction. Just seeing that this was his true fear created some release and breathing room. We would go further in the Healing Phase with the whole concept of sin and damnation versus God as unconditionally loving. (Instilling fear to curb negative behavior comes at grave price. Pun intended.)

The Laundry List

Throughout the Discovery Phase, I write down each negative self concept and belief that we uncover. I call this "the laundry list"—because Core Healing will only be complete when each of them has been replaced with its positive opposite. A positive opposite is essential. A behavioral void needs filling in order to focus the individual in a helpful direction. Plus, a positive opposite ensures that along side hundreds of other positives, together they become a mighty foundation for confident, wholesome conduct and purposeful direction.

In this process, we also look at what clients want their positives to be—what qualities, conditions, self concepts and beliefs they want to put in place. This is important as well. I worked with one woman who was always with men who were consumed by their work, spent very little time at home, and didn't pay as much attention to her as she would like. We carefully constructed a list of all the qualities she wanted in a man to whom she would like to be attracted. Sure enough, within a year she had met the perfect man. The one thing we had forgotten to include was "healthy." Tragically, he was ill and died just a year after they got together. The next time we worked together, we put "healthy" on the list.

Before exiting the Discovery Phase, I bear in mind all the information gathered during the intake interview. During the intake interview, I ask each client, "What is the worst thing you've ever done?" If a woman does not mention abortion, I ask, "Have you ever had an abortion?" I have found that many women who have had abortions have some level of "I deserve to be punished" operative in their subconscious and need to forgive themselves. Some women are fine with it, but others carry a self concept of "I'm a murderer." I ask the question to make sure we deal with that powerful negative self concept if it is in place.

During the entire Discovery process, I take verbatim notes—not just on what the client's negative self concepts and beliefs are, but on the words he or she actually uses to talk about the circumstances of their development (Bandler & Grinder, 1981). That way, during the Healing Phase, I can create a compassionate template that resonates with the client by using their own words, as well as be as accurate as possible.

THE HEALING PHASE

The Healing Phase immediately follows the Discovery Phase. All the data and information gleaned in the Discovery Phase is orchestrated into various types of healing: relational; emotional; physical; spiritual; and, behavioral. The total procedure usually takes about two and a half hours. A typical number of issues a person identifies for therapy is sixty. Many in the group of problems are interrelated. To deal with them all, generally takes about two to three of these two and a half hour sessions.

The Healing Phase must, of course, be done in hypnosis, so that we have access to the subconscious. This is what makes it possible to replace so many negative self concepts and beliefs so quickly. The subconscious simply does not argue. If, in the context of what was uncovered, we tell it to replace "I'm unlovable" with "I am lovable," it's done!

The process goes quickly for many reasons. First, we are only reconstructing negative self concepts and beliefs. Obviously, we want to keep and honor the positive. We are also working only with changes the client has chosen to make, and the client is viewed as a team player. We are also dealing only with the truth, and that creates an environment of ease and flow. Fixing problems becomes easy once you have the client's internal sense of the whole truth about themselves even if the truth, paradoxically, is false.

During the Healing Phase, we use many types of psychotherapeutic tools, all of which are respected and endorsed by my colleagues. These psychotherapeutic methods were developed by my predecessors. None were created by me. My contribution is not relinquishing the work of any one of these giants in the field of psychology in favor of but one or two of the latest methods. My work stands upon all their shoulders. My unique contribution is weaving them into the powerful, comprehensive process, based on the seminal process I experienced herein referred to as Core Healing. Some aspects of the following therapies are used: Cognitive Therapy (Beck); Direct Decision Making Therapy (Greenwald);

The Therapy of Logical Consequences (Dreikurs); Living by Choice (Tyrell); Cognitive Behavior Therapy (Ellis); Inner Child Work (Bradshaw and Riese); Neurolinguistic Programming (Erickson); Logotherapy (Frankl); and, Transactional Analysis (Berne). The work of Gardner regarding the issue of excellence as a goal versus perfection is important to mention here as well. (Perfectionism, as in having to do everything just right sometimes even to the extent of being insensitive and unkind in the process, is suffered by at least eighty percent of my clients. Perfectionism becomes a dis-ease process resulting in procrastination, indecisiveness, sleeplessness, anxiety, depression, and, at its worst, tyrannical parenting.)

Visualization - Setting the Stage

Imagine being in an empty theater resting comfortably in a center isle seat facing the stage. You, the reader, are the only one in the audience. You have been given this special invitation to witness what for some feels like a miracle. You are there to witness the setting of the stage. You are there to witness all those from The Discovery Phase coming onto the stage and interacting in such a way that produces core level healing for the one seeking help.

The concert master walks into the theater ready to orchestrate. He carries his sheaf of notes under his arm and carefully lays them out upon his stand. Everything that he requires to orchestrate the proceedings are there in the wings. All is in readiness awaiting his instruction to begin.

The lights in the theater dim. You hunker down ready to witness a unique action play, a symphony of orchestration. Themes of forgiveness will be interwoven with new understandings, making wiser choices, existing within oneself with loving kindness and with others in a bond of unconditional type loving.

Now, the concert master speaks an instruction into his lapel microphone. It is almost as if his very voice brings a stream of light rays raining down upon the stage from its rafters. Enlightened, the stage is now clear to see.

How the stage is set will depend on the client's choice of where this healing phase is to take place. Who all the players are will depend on which aged selves surfaced in The Discovery Phase. Those traumatized younger selves enter the stage. They await the adult self of today. Then, the perpetrators of the traumas that surfaced in the Discovery Phase arrive and stand before the injured selves.

Later, supportive cast may be brought in depending on the Spiritual direction from the client.

The progress of this orchestral work, this drama, is generally the same. The endings are similar, the crescendo potentially transcendent.

This symphonic orchestration has five basic aspects to its composition, unlike the traditional symphony that has four. Each movement is toward a type of healing - the healing of: relationships; emotional dis-ease; self defeating behavior; physical problems; and, any Spiritual issues. The following are highlights about what psychotherapeutic methods are used to orchestrate the core healing outcome.

Relationship Healing

Transactional Analysis is the therapy of choice here. Transactional Analysis (TA) is a social psychology developed by Eric Berne, M.D. It is a powerful tool that uses adult-to-adult communication to sort out relationships in a safe, mutually respectful, "I'm okay, you're okay" environment. Typically, TA is done with the conscious mind—but I have found that using it in hypnosis not only heals and resolves old traumatic events and relationships, but also gives people a template for adult-to-adult, assertive, resolution and compassion oriented behaviors, conversations, and interactions in the future. We use speaking to the person involved in the original traumatic incident as a way both to heal that trauma and replace the associated negative self concepts or beliefs, and also as a model for mature, compassionate, future interactions with that person.

In the Healing Phase, under hypnosis, I speak for the client to the mother, father, care giver, perpetrator, teacher, whoever precipitated the trauma. These conversations are respectful and reasoned, adult-to-adult interactions. They tell the other person exactly what happened, from the client's perspective, and make it clear that their behavior was unacceptable. There is honor and forgiveness, and the client leaves the situation feeling heard, understood, and respected. (In the beginning, I tried allowing clients to initiate these conversations themselves. The problem was that many have a "tyrant self" within, and they wound up saying things like, "You idiot! Why did you make that dumb decision? It's cost us grief all our life!" Because they weren't yet healed, they were still speaking from the old negative self concepts and beliefs. And since they were speaking to the subconscious, under hypnosis, whatever they said got imprinted and just reinforced the old beliefs! You can't have "an idiot" running this process. It's like having a client do their own open heart surgery. Just because they can hold a scalpel doesn't mean you let them do the cutting.)

Here is how TA might work in the Healing Phase. Jack got along beautifully with everyone at work except his boss, Ted, who was a powerful, pushy guy. Often when Ted started acting "overbearing," Jack found himself overreacting, pushing back, being aggressive rather than assertive, and trying to one-up Ted to "show him he can't push me around." Jack was raised in a home where he was often ordered around and told what to do by his father. He felt controlled and dominated, and usually just gave in and complied. The only times he ever got his way were when, older, he put up a terrible fight and forced his dad to back off. When he was around Ted at work, especially when Ted was acting forcefully or asserting his role of "boss," Jack felt almost dizzy. He overreacted and pushed back hard—just as he had with his father. It had gotten to the point that one of them was going to have to go.

TA was a perfect tool to use with Jack. Under hypnosis, I spoke for Jack to his father, adult-to-adult. "Jack" said, "You know, Dad, when I was a kid and you always made my decisions for me, I either had to rebel or do what you told me to do. Now I find myself either letting people control me, or rebelling in ways that are inappropriate. I want you to know that I'm not going to slide into that position anymore. I'm going to stand up for myself, but I don't have to shout or get nasty about it. I am a grown man, and have the wherewithal to state my position. I don't have to be overwhelmed by someone else's strong position, as I did when I was a child."

Since we are in the presence of Jack's subconscious, we are giving him a whole new imprint for how to handle people like Ted, people who had elicited from him the same childlike reaction as he had to his father. Thus, if someone else who is pushy and forceful or even strongly assertive crosses Jack's path, he now has imprinted a mature calm way of responding to such an individual. Now, in adult and constructive fashion, he has the "experience" to smoothly handle matters. In addition, and when appropriate, he also has been imprinted with the skill to engage in co-creative, problem solving dialogue.

Behavior Correction

In the Healing Phase, the adult self is positioned as the wise parent of the traumatized selves that are in need of core healing. Sometimes, the child selves had rather toxic parents or situations affecting them and they are in need of reparenting. The self of today has to be imprinted with the mantle of wisdom, the "good" parent, the unconditionally loving one. Another way of viewing the situation is the adult self is taking over as team captain. The adult self becomes the captain/coach. He conveys the voice and skill of the concert master (the therapist) to bring the various sections (the other selves) into harmony. That therapeutic voice, vested with healing experience, gently instills healing concepts. Their history is viewed for what it was—something over which they had no control. The negative effects of that history are reframed with a vision of new possibilities for the now and the future. The themes, spoken of earlier, are played out in the form of a discussion. How the negative self concepts and beliefs came to be are put in the context of the traumas discussed in the Discovery Phase. Then, better concepts are suggested to be implemented now. One by one, the negative self concepts and beliefs are discussed. Positive opposites are suggested for the replacement of each one. It is the choice of the whole team as to whether or not to act in concert based on the new ways of thinking about themselves. (The TA work done earlier, in part, has given a context for the relinquishment of the old ideas about self.)

During this reframing work a variety of psychotherapeutic techniques come into play. Key dis-ease words used by the client to describe their condition are brought into focus and rethought. (Neuro Linguistic Programming) Inner child work is conducted. Responsibility taking is modeled. Living by choice without fearing failure or making a mistake is encouraged. They become instead, a wise person. A wise person does not fear mistakes or failure—they are those who learn from them. The positive consequences of making wiser choices are looked at. New decisions about self are made. Living in the new now is envisioned. Success is now doable with the beliefs about self that are ready to more consistently attract wonderful opportunities into their lives (Byrne, 2006).

Emotional Healing

The wise adult self deals with the mistaken ideas accumulated about themselves and how they affected them emotionally. Then too, the core fears as self concepts are therapeutically discussed as well. It is all part and parcel of the corrective reframing.

Physical Healing

Healing the body, atypically, is conducted during the Discovery Phase. When the physical dis-ease began, which is brought out in the Discovery Phase, that self is dealt with right then and there. A comforting, compassionate, forgiving environment is created. Various healing visualizations are brought into play. (Siegel, 1986) The creativity of the therapist gets free rein. Negative self concepts and beliefs that created the dis-ease predicament are corrected. The healing is visualized as accomplished even though the amount of time the subconscious deems appropriate for the particular malady to be resolved may be left open.

Spiritual Healing

The stage empties through the various healing aspects of this concert. The cast of characters leave one by one as dialogue between the adult self and each of them is concluded. Then, when there is consensus among the selves for their newly sculpted self to take charge, they become one with that adult self. They are integrated back into the adult self. Thus, the stage is now cleared except for the adult self. The wise self, that adult self stands center stage and is ensconced in the rays of light. The final act is at hand. The client's Prayer comes into play. A realization of that person's blessings are emphasized - an opportunity for the personal communication of thanks with the unconditionally loving Parent provided. The client's prayer becomes the template for Spiritual interaction and integration. It is also an opportunity to instill Oprah Winfrey's saving grace "staying in an attitude of gratitude."

Bringing their enlightenment with them, their new decisions to guide them, the client is reoriented to the actual time and place and is brought out of the state of hypnosis. The symphony is now alive in the mind of the individual even though that particular concert is over.

CLEANING HOUSE AND DUSTING

This initial series of sessions—in which we delete and replace all the negatives the client and I can identify at the time—is what I call "Cleaning House." We deal systematically with each negative self concept or belief associated with the problems that he or she presented, using the process described in this chapter.

But suppose someone came to Core Healing for eating that was out of control. They complete Cleaning House, but three weeks later find themselves in front of a pastry case, staring at an apple fritter and struggling not to succumb. It may be that while Cleaning House, we discovered, deleted and replaced fourteen of the twenty negative self concepts and beliefs in the constellation that governed their relationship with food. They feel a definite improvement, but they want to come back and deal with those six remaining negatives that are making it difficult for them to completely embrace their healthy relationship with food. They may not know what these negatives are, or even how many of them there are—but they sense that some are left and want to get rid of them, and so schedule a visit. After all, the siren call of the apple fritter said, "get moving."

I call what is done during that visit "Dusting." As a now savvy, experienced client, we can team up to uncover the rest of those "suckers." "Suckers" are what I call negative self concepts and beliefs.

While we remove as many negatives as we can when "Cleaning House," some negatives may remain dormant for a different reason, a reason other than they were not found the first time around. A subsequent event, like a thirty-ninth birthday or the death of a particular person, may "awaken" those negatives. When surfaced in response to the event the negative(s), create dis-ease. The dis-ease would likely take the form of anxiety and/or depression.

For some people, Core Healing seems to be "time-released." Ellen told me she was complete with all of her issues and "Why?" questions when we finished—yet she said that in the following months, she wasn't sure our work had made any real difference. She called me a year later to say, "I wasn't sure you had really helped me, but it has dawned on me you cured me of depression—and it feels like *forever*!" Sometimes the shift is so subtle that it takes awhile for people to recognize it. Other people don't *feel* very different, and are surprised when they see themselves *behaving* so differently—not engaging in negative behaviors or relationships, and doing good things for themselves like exercising and eating well. The shifts occur so naturally, it is as if the "new" self has always been that way.

In these first six chapters, we have looked at what Core Healing is and how it works. In Part 2, we will explore how it works with specific dis-eases.

PART 2

The chapters that follow discuss how Core Healing can be applied to various dis-eases of our times. Our discussions of these conditions are not meant to be exhaustive, by any means. Rather, they are meant to give a glimpse into how Core Healing might be used in that situation. Many excellent texts provide a fuller view of each of these dis-eases.

As you will see, these dis-eases often overlap, as do the negative self concepts and beliefs that are at their roots. And as we have said before, there is no strict correlation between specific negatives and particular dis-eases. We will list negative self concepts and beliefs commonly held by people with a particular condition, but these are not the only negatives that can be at the root, and each of these negatives may also manifest contributory to another dis-ease.

Chapter 7

DEPRESSION

Depression has reached epidemic proportions in the United States. An op-ed piece in *The New York Times* notes:

> "Depression is the leading cause of disability worldwide, according to the World Health Organization. It costs more in treatment and lost productivity than anything but heart disease. Suicide is the 11th most common cause of death in the United States, claiming 30,000 lives each year. Despite medical advances in the last 20 years that have greatly improved our ability to help those who suffer from depression, we lack an effective system for administering care. Only a very small percentage of depressives who seek help receive appropriate treatment for their condition…many sufferers are left to spiral, unsupported, into despair…"

> "Our Great Depression," by Andrew Solomon,
> *The New York Times*, November 17, 2006

WHAT IS DEPRESSION?

Depression is an emotional state, caused by negative self concepts and beliefs that generalize into feelings of sadness, lack of energy or motivation, being tired, resentment, and often a sense of despair. While the basics of depression are similar for each person, depression can look different on each of us because we each can have somewhat varying constellations of self concepts and beliefs.

One of the, if not the most common undercurrent for depression is anger. Not everyone is aware of feeling angry when they are depressed, but anger is one of the most critical components of depression for most, if not all, people. The anger can be about anything—not having what they want, not being as smart about something as they thought they should have been, being out of control, that the world is not a better place, etc.

The worst kind of anger generative of depression is anger with oneself. One result is enervating rage, anger that has no place to go but repetitively, exhaustively inward.

Contributive types of anger can be about not being able to find a job and feed the children, about not having the money to retire, about not finding a mate, about the loss of a person or condition that defined us, or about anything that makes us feel out of control, helpless, and a negative self concept of being hopeless. The progression, without intervention, is from helpless, to hopeless, to despair. At its worst, despair moves toward suicide. We just don't know what else to do, and conclude, "I might as well be dead." (At least causing my own death is one thing I can control.)

People who are depressed often experience the condition of living with little or no pleasure. They don't believe that they are supposed to have pleasure in their lives, and abandon the part of themselves that plays and enjoys, if they even ever knew how. They often adopt the self concept, "I'm a workaholic." Depression can also affect eating—whether they overeat for comfort, or whether they refuse to eat, exacerbating their lack of energy.

People describe their experience of depression as feeling: helpless, unmotivated, angry, grief stricken, anxious, guilty, sad/unhappy, out of control, hopeless, and powerless. They often say things like:
- "I have always been sad, lazy and seen my life as meaningless."
- "I feel spiritually disconnected."
- "I give up easily, and feel like a failure."
- "I have always felt there was something wrong with me. I've had thoughts of suicide to rid myself of the pain and grief, and the fear that I would never get better."
- "I am afraid of change and of being wrong, and angry with myself for being wrong so much of the time."
- "My feelings are easily hurt. It is difficult for me to accept help from others, and at the same time I can't say 'No' when people ask me to do things."
- "A part of me wants to stay depressed. I use the emotional pain as punishment for not living the life I was supposed to live. Without the punishment, I'd be even less disciplined."
- "Nothing I do is good enough. I can't relax and enjoy life. If I'm not doing

everything perfectly, I don't feel like I deserve to be happy."

These statements clearly reflect the negative self concepts and beliefs that give rise to depression.

We often hear that depression is caused by chemical imbalances. We also hear that the chemical imbalances are caused by depression. As already noted, I believe the answer to the "Which came first, the chicken or the egg?" question is that negative self concepts and beliefs came first. They generated the depression, which can then affect a change in chemistry. We know that negative thoughts can actually change our physiology, and I believe that this is what happens in the case of depression. Negative self concepts and beliefs can lead to feeling out of control, which can lead to despair, which can depress serotonin levels, which can exacerbate feelings of depression.

DEPRESSION AS A LEARNED BEHAVIOR

Children are like sponges; they absorb whatever is around them and very quickly. They learn ways of thinking and ways of behaving that neither they nor their parents are necessarily aware that they are learning.

How to become depressed is something we learn when we are very young. When children see their parents being depressed—and becoming more depressed in response to particular stimuli like the kids starting school, spouses going on business trips, losing a job, feeling out of control of their predicaments, or simply as a way to get attention—they absorb the message, "This is an appropriate way to be in the world, and an appropriate response to certain situations.

Children learn by example. They learn when to get depressed, when to get more depressed, and how to get depressed. They absorb the thought patterns, the beliefs that produce depression. Same sex patterning is based on this is what males or this is what females do under such and such circumstances. Some patterning may well be undifferentiated in this way. Depression as an attention getter is also learned. "Oh, poor thing, she is always so unhappy." Depression becomes like a bad habit.

Children learn depression from their parents in many ways. Most people are excited about being parents, and want to do the best possible job—but we have seen that if they want to be perfect parents, then they must have perfect children! When the child brings home a report card with four A's and one B, the

B gets all the attention and the child gets the message, "I'm not good enough." The children of "perfect parents" often hear things like, "You mean you're wearing those slacks with that shirt? Hmm. I thought I taught you how to coordinate better." The stress of needing to be perfect is enormous. The child's anxiety feeds on the absorption of more anxiety producing negative self concepts and beliefs. When this happens anxiety can become chronic. Depression follows based on feeling so out of control.

Another way that parents inadvertently foster depression is by doing everything for their children. They say, "No, that's okay. I'll take care of it. I'll do it." We have seen that when parents do this, children don't learn basic life skills. The parents are overly helpful with homework, give the child money without the child having to earn or organize it, clean the child's room, and protect him or her from any social discomfort. Either the parents or "the help" do all the cleaning, laundry, cooking, and bill-paying. When children find themselves in the position of needing those skills, they are lost. They don't have the fundamentals for survival in our society. The result? As adults, they don't know how to cope with life and fear going out into the world. Their minds are filled with frantic thoughts of, "I just don't know how to do this," "I don't know how to get along, how to get by." Again, the result can be significant anxiety that courts depression.

Another difficulty for people with depression is that they feel they don't know how to be happy because they have never *been* happy. I remind them that they have witnessed people being happy, and so that imprint is in their minds. All they have to do is live out the imprint. Imitate it until it becomes them.

ROOTS OF DEPRESSION

Depression can result from any or all of the following:
1. Intense anger at self, which leads to abandoning ourselves as a form of self punishment, which can lead to addictions, suffocating our own success, lack of self care, and a variety of other negative outcomes
2. Feeling out of control, the result of unabated anxiety, which occurs when nothing we try is working, when we feel cornered and trapped, and we can't pinpoint the source of the anxiety
3. Feelings of helpless and/or powerlessness, leading to a sense of despair
4. Being labeled as "depressed"

5. "Needing" to be depressed in order to acquire some secondary gain, or using "being depressed" as a way to manipulate or control others

Again, the belief that "I deserve to be abandoned (by myself, others, and/or God)" is a powerful negative force. Many issues "peel down" to this core belief. Supposed I lose my favorite uncle. I am grief stricken, but suppose the depression lingers and deepens over the months or years. I might say, "My grief reaction is all out of proportion. Yes, I loved him, but he was 90 and had lived a good life. I knew he was going to die. Why, two years later, am I still depressed?"

This would be one of the "Why?" questions in the Discovery Phase of Core Healing. It might get "peeled down" through a series of questions to the real reason for the grief.

Question: What does it mean that your uncle is gone?
Answer: I'm afraid.
Question: And what are you afraid of?
Answer: That I'll be alone. He was the only one in my corner and now he's gone.
Question: And what would it mean if you were alone?
Answer: I'd be completely abandoned because no one else in my family was there for me.
Question: And what would happen if you were completely abandoned?
Answer: If I get sick or in trouble, there will be no one to care for me and I'll die.

So the grief was not just situational grief over my uncle's death, but a core fear of abandonment with no one there to care for me which, unabated, slid into depression. The Healing Phase would take me, in hypnosis, through a process of realizing that there is someone there for me and will always be—if only myself and/or God. (When we get down to the fear of death, the fear of the unknown, it is difficult to achieve absolute comfort and confidence without some spiritual sense of connection.)

Anxiety is another strong root of depression. Anxiety, unchecked, leads inevitably to depression. Many people have a dual diagnosis of anxiety and depression. It is not uncommon for someone to have a significant anxiety problem and be diagnosed as depressed, because you can't help but feel depressed if you are feeling anxious all the time. Anxiety, a cadre of fears that are severe and chronic, leads to feeling out of control—and that is a primary source of feeling depressed. The more negative self concepts and beliefs are involved, the longer they have gone on, and the more severe they are, the deeper the depression. The greater the intensity and duration of the anxiety, and the more out of control people feel, the more depressed they become.

COMMON NEGATIVE SELF CONCEPTS AND BELIEFS

In the Discovery Phase of Core Healing, I make lists of each client's constellations of negative self concepts and beliefs. Below are some of the most common among people who come to me for depression:

- "I do most things wrong." "I feel so helpless." "I must be a hopeless case."
- "There is something wrong with me."
- "I'm to blame when others abandon me."
- "It's not a good thing to have fun."
- "I deserve to be abandoned."
- "I deserve to be punished."
- "I am angry with myself and deserve to be severely punished for my mistakes."
- "Punishment is good as a way to enforce discipline."
- "I can't relax and enjoy life. I have to be perfect."
- "I abandoned my creative passion."
- "I am winding up alone, without any close friends."
- "I couldn't take the disappointment of being left again."
- "I'm afraid of pain and being hurt."
- "I don't have a right to be happy."

DEPRESSION FOR SECONDARY GAIN

Depression is very often used for secondary gain. We talked about secondary gain in Chapter 3, as a way to manipulate people into giving us something we want without actually having to ask for it directly. When we don't have the social skills or the freedom to ask for what we want—a hug, a cup of tea, attention—we can often bring people running by being, or acting, depressed.

We aren't always aware that we are using depression, or an illness as another example, for secondary gain. This is what some of my clients said after they realized what they were doing:

- "Depression is a way to get physical closeness without having to ask for it. I'm afraid of rejection when I express my neediness. But when I'm depressed, my husband always holds me."
- "When I'm depressed, I don't have to do anything for anybody. I don't have to perform. I can let down the burden of having to make my mother happy—and I don't have to be responsible for her feelings."
- "I was sickly as a child and I enjoyed my hospital stays. I liked the physical and emotional feeling of being taken care of. Now I use depression to get those same feelings."

Some people act depressed, even when they aren't, in order to get some secondary gain. They get a clear benefit from being depressed—sympathy, attention, being taken care of, etc.—and so it becomes second nature. Bob thought of himself as the man of the house and wanted to support his wife and children, but he had little education and few vocational skills. When he became "depressed," he could go on Medicaid and Social Security in order to support his household.

Many people use depression to manipulate their spouses. Jeff had it down to a science. He didn't like to go out and socialize. He much preferred to stay home and be a couch potato. But his wife liked going out and was always on his case. "All you want to do is sit home," she would say. "Can't we go out and spend the evening with friends sometimes? I'd like to go to the movies. How about going to dinner?" But Jeff just "couldn't get it together" to join her because he was depressed. He even went to a doctor and got a diagnosis and a prescription to support his claim. He had a disease, for heaven's sake! Couldn't she just leave him alone?

Sometimes people use depression for extreme secondary gain. We've talked about the danger of the words, "I can't handle it." They are often an indication that people want a "mental vacation," and will do just about anything to get it—including "going crazy." We all know how to look and act crazy. And if we've made a conscious decision that is in harmony with the subconscious to take a mental vacation, that means we need to get someone to take care of us.

There are two basic institutions in our society that guarantee they will take care of us: jails and mental health facilities. Given these options, the self concepts of each individual will choose the particular facility. And once they get admitted, their responsibility for self is considerably, if not totally, diminished. They are given food, a bed, medications, and people to care for their every need. The most serious consequence of "not being able to handle it" is, of course, suicide.

FORGIVENESS, REVISITED

The most common, and most powerful, cause of depression is anger with ourselves. This is why forgiveness—the letting go of pain and anger that we discussed in Chapters 1 and 5—is an enormous step toward healing depression. That forgiveness needs to include forgiveness of ourselves, others, and God.

We are taught as children that punishment is good, that it "evens the score," mitigates bad behavior, and is the inevitable result of doing something wrong. Since nobody goes through life without making mistakes and doing things that are wrong, almost everyone has the self concept "I deserve to be punished." We carry that with us for decades, and sometimes for a lifetime. Relinquishing that self concept combined with forgiveness is the only solution.

Forgiveness also helps alleviate the fear of being abandoned. It is possible that "I deserve to be abandoned" is at the heart of our depression epidemic. We saw in the discussion of abandonment in Chapter 4 that people usually do not relate to this core fear—but that, in fact, most people do have an "I deserve to be abandoned" belief being actualized, to some degree.

CASE STUDY: Sandy

Sandy suffered from severe depression. She had done cognitive therapy with minimal results, and didn't want to start anti-depressants. She didn't know where to turn, and a friend recommended Core Healing.

Sandy was always tired. Her friends told her, "You have to get out of the house!" But she always made excuses. During what she called the "dark times," she couldn't leave the bed or the couch. She didn't exercise, barely had enough energy to get to work, and when she got home collapsed in front of CNN with a big bowl of chocolate pudding with whipped cream. She cried a great deal, drank more than she thought was healthy, and was sixty pounds overweight. Sandy had had learning disabilities as a child and had been left back in school. Despite this, she continued in school and became a dental hygienist—but the depression was always lurking in the background, playing havoc with the physical, emotional, spiritual, behavioral, and relational aspects of her life.

In the Discovery Phase, she remembered being told by a trusted teacher, "You'll never amount to anything!" This incident, and subsequent reinforcing events, led to a constellation of negative self concepts that included:

- "I'm not good enough."
- "My opinion doesn't count."
- "I'm worthless."
- "I can't love or trust myself."
- "I'll never do anything of consequence with my life."
- "Don't make waves."
- "You'll never make it on your own."
- "I'm unlovable."

One by one, we deleted these negative self concepts and beliefs and replaced them with concepts that built confidence, serenity, happiness, and positive self care. I talked with Sandy recently, four years after our work together. This is what she said:

> *The depression is gone! I sometimes get depressed over a death or something that is genuinely sad, but I know how to deal with it. It doesn't take me over. Plus, I can take care of myself in life, and I never really believed I could. It's hard even to imagine that I thought those things about myself!*
>
> *I still work hard, but I have incredible energy. I just laugh more. I used to cry a lot. I walk with my friends, and one of them told me the other day, "Wow, you have so much more energy!" I don't dwell anymore on the negative. I wake up every day and do yoga. I never did that! Then I stretch and meditate.*
>
> *My relationships are completely different. I used to avoid conflict with people. I'd say "Everything's good," even when it*

wasn't. Now I voice my opinion. I'm more honest. I don't hide away from people anymore. I have a lot of close friends and I see them more often now. My family sees a big change.

My food choices are different. I don't eat sugar, and I don't drink at all. I turned in the chocolate pudding with whipped cream for turnips and carrots.

The greatest gift of Core Healing is that I'm so much more relaxed and comfortable with myself. I love myself, which I never did. If things get tough I just tell myself, "Take a deep breath." Last evening in the parking lot at the dental office where I work, I left my keys in the car. Before, I would have gone ballistic. It would have been the end of the world. But I just said to myself, "Let's not make it into a big deal. Don't get down on yourself." Before, I would have said, "What a dummy!" Instead, I just called AAA and then called some friends while I waited, just to pass the time. I transformed the negative situation into something positive.

Bottom line, I just don't have the fears and guilt I used to have. I was driven by fear. Fear of people not believing in me, fear of my work, the fear of not being lovable, and of not being good enough. Now people call me to ask what I think. That to me is the greatest feeling. I was just going in to resolve depression. I didn't realize I would get all this!

Sandy was lucky in that she was single and did not have a partner who could have been an accomplice so to speak. Therefore, she didn't encounter one of the problems that often follows healing from depression.

When people have been depressed for a long time, they have often set up their lives based on their negative self concepts. Releasing those concepts, and replacing them with positives, can affect their relationships. For instance, they may have a partner who constantly delivers the message "You're not good enough." This has been consistent with their own subconscious beliefs, so it hasn't been a problem. But now that self concept is gone. It has been replaced by a positive self concept like, "I deserve to be respected and appreciated." Suddenly, the partner is saying things that are not okay—and is getting entirely new responses.

Understandably, this creates conflict. Everyone needs to get clear on the new ground rules, and take a good look at whether or not they can embrace them.

We don't have to live with depression, and most of us don't need to take depression medication to dull the symptoms. There is another way to deal with this debilitating condition, a way that frees us to love ourselves, one another, and feel empowered.

Chapter 8
ANXIETY

Anxiety is another dis-ease that is epidemic in our society. One reason is that both the anxious feelings people experience, and the associated physical symptoms like high blood pressure, are medicated with drugs. We never get to the root of the problem—the negative self concepts and beliefs—and so the anxiety is not dissolved nearly as often as we would all like to see.

Anxiety and depression are brother and sister. The more anxious a person becomes, the more likely that anxiety will expand into depression. Depression can exist without anxiety, but anxiety that is left to simmer in negative thinking seems to court depression.

Like depression, anxiety is quite often a learned behavior. When I ask people under hypnosis, "From whom did you learn to anxiety (worry)?" the answer is always immediate. "My mother," "My father," "My Uncle Bill." We can learn to do nervous.

Anxiety disorders also stem from agitating in utero experience. They also occur in response to postponed bonding after birth. These sources can leave a person with what has been described as free floating anxiety.

Regardless of the sources for anxiety, there is one caveat. The client, as they are freed from their core fears, must be absolutely, unequivocally dedicated to averting "stinkin' thinkin'." I teach them the importance, and the how of doing this. If a client does not do what is instructed, this heedlessness needs to become an issue for therapy because if they won't be strict in the formation of a new habit of thinking positively, they can readily reinfect themselves.

WHAT IS ANXIETY?

Anxiety is characterized by uneasy feelings, persistent worry and fear, inability to relax, nervousness, difficulty sleeping, restlessness, and anticipating the worst. Anxiety disorder is an umbrella term that ranges from severe stress to panic attacks, phobic reactions, generalized anxiety, and can result in obsessive compulsive behavior in various forms such as rituals, addictions, etc. Like all emotions, anxiety has various levels of intensity. If there is no intervention, anxiety leads to feelings of being out of control, which lead to depression and an intense desire to escape.

For anxiety to exist, four things must be present:
1. *Negative self concepts and beliefs capable of eliciting fear.*
2. *A trigger that surfaces a relevant negative constellation. The trigger is a thought or thoughts derived while reflectively trancing out or when faced with a particular situation, present or anticipated.*
3. *Supportive, fear based, conscious thoughts that galvanize and expand the anxiety reaction.*
4. *A fear of fear*

Panic Attacks

Panic attacks are a frequent manifestation of anxiety. The *Diagnostic and Statistical Manual (Fourth Edition)* identifies several criteria for panic attacks, and says that if four of them are present and peak within ten minutes, an individual can be considered to have had a panic attack. These criteria are:
1. Palpitations, pounding heart, or accelerated heart rate
2. Sweating
3. Trembling or shaking
4. Sensations of shortness of breath or smothering
5. A feeling of choking
6. Chest pain or discomfort
7. Nausea or abdominal distress
8. Feeling dizzy, unsteady, lightheaded, or faint
9. Derealization (feelings of unreality) or depersonalization (being detached from oneself)
10. Fear of losing control or going crazy
11. Fear of dying
12. Paresthesias (numbness or tingling sensations)
13. Chills or hot flashes

Pouring Gas on the Fire

Feeling occasional anxiety is different from experiencing a full blown panic attack, or from allowing anxiety to become severe or chronic. We all have constellations supportive of our fears, and those fears often get triggered—but in order for the fears to mushroom into a panic attack, or into chronic or severe anxiety, it is helpful in a sardonic sense to throw gasoline on the fire. We do this with the thoughts generated by our negative self concepts and beliefs. These reactions accumulate, build, and produce higher and higher levels of anxiety either immediately or over time.

They sound like this:

- "Oh, I'm getting another panic attack. I wonder how many I'm gonna get. This is getting worse! I'm getting more and more anxious. Now my heart is pounding, and I can't breathe!"
- "I never get anything right. I can't even do normal things without getting panicky. And once it starts, I can't stop it!"
- "I am feeling more and more out of control, like a train without any brakes."

With anxiety, we are dealing with "fight or flight" hormones. In order to avoid giving ourselves over to "fight" or "flight," we need tools. We need to stop pouring gas on the fire with negative thinking and develop new habits. Instead of berating ourselves for being anxious or "about to have a panic attack," we need to learn to say to ourselves, "I know how to take control. This will pass. I'll work it out. I may be a little uncomfortable at the moment, but it'll pass."

The language with which to take constructive control of how one feels must be taught. To conquer anxiety, as one example of discomforting emotion, a person must memorize some basic positive self statements like those in the foregoing paragraph, to be immediately retrieved when fear is felt. The client must tenaciously apply them. It is not a time for sloppiness. Victory depends on preparedness. One client who took this lesson to heart, did his homework so as to be ready to apply the self statements whenever needed. He said to me, "I am so happy to be able finally to rid myself of an anxiety attack, I almost look forward to the next one." Instead of running from, or stuffing down, medicating, or blowing off fear with anger, he was now free to take conscious control. This freedom was within reach because the core fears that were haunting him had been removed and replaced with positives. It was wonderful to witness his relief at being so capable at dousing the conflagration called anxiety attacks. Without this type of teamwork victory would be temporary at best and ever so elusive at worst.

THE SPIRITUAL DIMENSION OF ANXIETY

Anxiety is one of the most obviously fear-based dis-eases. In order to be anxious, our fears need to be triggered. Most of these fears ultimately "peel down" to fear of death or more precisely, being terrified of dying. The final question is often, "And what would happen if you were to die?"

As we have noted, people with some idea of the Divine or of an afterlife are more likely to have an answer to that question. Their answers may differ widely from Heaven to burning in hell. Even if they do not articulate any awareness of what happens after death, if they choose to view God as benevolent and unconditionally loving, it is a comfort to them to know that they are in such Hands. When people have no sense of the Divine, eternalness, or a benevolent embracing deity, sometimes the best that can then be offered is the existential choice: "You can either be afraid of dying, or not." At this juncture, their homework of writing a prayer is an essential guide for the therapist.

COMMON NEGATIVE SELF CONCEPTS AND BELIEFS

When people come to Core Healing to alleviate anxiety, some of their most common "Why?" questions are:
- Why do I feel out of control in my life?
- Why do I feel worthless, not good enough, not attractive enough?
- Why am I jealous?
- Why do I sometimes act like a fake?
- Why do I smoke?
- Why do I get nauseous when going out with people?
- Why do I need constant validation?
- Why do I feel intimidated?
- Why do I feel so alone?
- Why am I shy?
- Why don't I like myself?
- Why do I feel insecure?
- Why do I have anxiety attacks?
- Why don't I trust anyone?

Some core fears that often trigger anxiety are the fears of abandonment, of being alone and unwanted (an outcast), of dying alone, of the unknown, of humiliation, of being stupid, of being unlovable, of having to compete, of failing, and of having to be responsible for one's life.

As we have said, any combination of negative self concepts and beliefs can produce any dis-ease. However, these are the kinds of negatives that often occur for people with anxiety:

- "I don't deserve to be happy."
- "I'm helpless."
- "I don't fit in."
- "I'm rebellious."
- "I am bad."
- "I'm a fake."
- "I'm defective."
- "I am not supposed to be in control of myself (my mother, or father, or husband is)."
- "I am skeptical."
- "I'm impatient."
- "I'm a girl, not a woman."
- "I can't depend on anyone to look out for me."
- "I deserve to be abandoned by the man in my life."
- "I don't like myself because my dad wished I'd been a boy."
- "I deserve to be punished."
- "I have to hurt others to alleviate my own pain."
- "I don't trust anybody."
- "I'm sad."
- "I have to protect myself from pain by acting mean, hiding away from people, pushing them away, and making them feel sorry for me."
- "I have to get sick to get attention."
- "I'm not attractive."
- "I'm inferior."
- "I'm weak."
- "I'm a worry wart."
- "I have to make people feel sorry for me."
- "Sex is taboo."

- "God is scary."
- "Worry protects me from death."
- "I am not at all lovable."
- "Other people are better than I am."
- "Women deserve to be abused."
- "You need to act mean to defend yourself."
- "I am unsafe when alone."
- "I constantly wonder when my next anxiety attack will come."
- "I'm really losing control."
- "I'm afraid I will be like this forever."
- "Responsibility is scary (being at fault)."
- "I deserve to be condemned."

CASE STUDY: Lori

To everyone around her, Lori's life looked perfect. She was married to a man she loved, had two beautiful children who were both old enough to be in school, and had just gone back to work part time as a teacher. Her twenty-hour work week was manageable, and her mother helped out with the kids—but Lori had started having panic attacks at school. She had managed to cover them up so far, but didn't know how she could continue and was on the verge of quitting.

"What's the matter with you?" her mother said when Lori told her about the panic attacks. "You don't know how lucky you are!"

"You can do this, honey," her husband encouraged.

"I have all the support I could ever want," Lori told me. "I don't understand what's wrong with me, and why I'm so anxious and upset. The classes I'm teaching are easy, my mother picks up all the slack, and Don couldn't be more supportive. But I just get taken over by the anxiety. Then I start thinking about how terrible I am to react that way, and I get even more anxious."

It was a classic case of throwing gas on the fire. Her mother's explicit message was that there was something wrong with her. Then Lori berates herself for feeling unreasonable anxiety. But before working with Lori to develop more positive responses, we needed to discover and erase the negative self concepts and beliefs that were at the heart of her anxiety. Moreover, we had to delete the newly developed ones unwittingly implanted by her mother and by herself in reaction to her mother. (Remember, in a state of even the least bit of fear there is access to the subconscious mind.)

Under hypnosis, Lori recalled a time when she was in middle school. Within a week, she had gotten an award for the best grades. Later, she was elected "Queen" of the spring dance, as well as chosen captain of the soccer team. She reveled in all her successes, and had announced at the dinner table that Friday night, "I'm the best at everything!"

Her mother, with the best of intentions and simply wanting to save Lori from the resentment she might experience if she expressed herself that way to her peers, said, "Don't get too big for your britches. Nobody likes someone who thinks they have it all!"

Lori was crushed. In the panic that followed being publicly humiliated at the dinner table, what got imprinted on her subconscious was, "I can't have what I want, or people will hate me." There were many subsequent reinforcing events, and the constellation grew to include:

- "I don't deserve to have it all."
- "I'll be alone if I succeed."
- "People will abandon me if I excel."
- "I don't deserve to enjoy success."

With these negatives in place, the scenario in which she had a great marriage, great children in school, and a great job was quite threatening. It produced high levels of anxiety in Lori. By having panic attacks at work, she had been systematically jeopardizing her job so that she wouldn't "have it all."

We deleted these and other negatives, had Lori talk things through with her mother and others in her Cast of Characters, and replaced her negative self concepts and beliefs with such positives as:

- "I am free to enjoy 'having it all' yet feel ever grateful for my blessings."
- "Everyone supports my success."
- "I can let myself enjoy being at work and doing well."
- "I deserved to succeed in all I do."
- "There is nothing fundamentally wrong with me."
- "I now know how to handle myself upon an occasion when I feel afraid."

Lori learned to stop when she had a recollection of a panic attack, and use positive self talk to get over the fear the memory may have induced. She understood her tendency to throw gas on the fire, and took specific steps to avoid doing so. In her case, what worked was to keep a list of her positives in her purse. When she felt something uncomfortable surfacing, she simply found a private place, took a deep breath, read them over, and deliberately opened herself up to allowing in the pleasure of living the life of her dreams. Teaching clients such self control is essential.

These positive behaviors were effective because the negative self concepts and beliefs were gone. It's not that Lori will never experience anxiety again. We human beings are hard-wired to respond to fear with "flight or fight." It's a survival mechanism, and we need it to protect ourselves from genuine danger. But Lori can now make choices, and she has skills to manage anxiety rather than be paralyzed by it.

Chapter 9
STRESS MANAGEMENT

We now recognize that stress is a major contributor to both psychological and physical dis-ease. A certain amount of stress is inevitable. It is a natural by-product of life. But when stress spirals out of control, it has a negative impact on our relationships, emotions, physical wellbeing, spirituality, and behavior. This occurs when normal stress is fed by negative self concepts and beliefs, and mushrooms into anxiety, followed by depression.

With a combination of Core Healing and stress management tools, we can keep stress from snowballing into something that eats away at the quality of our lives.

STRESS: FEELING OUT OF CONTROL

The word *"stress"* is a euphemism for feeling out of control. Feeling out of control is scary. The more out of control we feel, the more fear we experience. If we feel completely out of control, we may experience *intense* fear, the kind of fear associated with feeling like one is going *crazy*

Using the euphemism of "stress" helps us cope with feeling out of control. Some symptoms of stress are feeling exhausted, grouchy, and frazzled. Life is no fun, we don't sleep well, and we can't seem to pull it together. At its worst, we can feel in dire predicament, as if we are in over our heads and have few, if any, options. As time goes on, such feelings can intensify. We can feel more and more stuck, more and more trapped in that predicament.

What is the difference between stress and anxiety? Basically, it is one of degree. On a scale of 0 – 7, with 0 being no anxiety and 7 being a full blown panic attack, stress would be a 3 – 5. Stress is a generalized sense of not being able to manage well enough. Anxiety is more intense, and characterized by feeling even more out of control. The level of stress a person experiences depends on the number and intensity of their negative self concepts and beliefs, and on the circumstances that trigger them. These negatives, in the absence of life and stress management skills, can lead to feelings of "hanging on by my fingertips."

People do not generally come into therapy with stress as their presenting problem. They are more likely to present problems such as substance abuse, overeating, anxiety attacks, depression, sleep problems, or problems with their spouse.

In some cases, diagnoses of ADD (Attention Deficit Disorder) and ADHD (Attention Deficit and Hyperactivity Disorder) are given to children and adults who are simply stressed out. Children who live in stressful homes are given medications and imprinted with the self concept that there is something wrong with them. They are "ADD" or "ADHD." That is how they begin to define themselves, and how others also come to define them. So the stressed circumstances at home, among their peers, with their teachers plus the labels facilitate the continuing manifestation of those symptoms, which reinforces the self concepts, "I am ADD" or "I am ADHD." Fostering further entrenchment in these self concepts are the additional ones birthed through the process of labeling. Some likely self concepts developed are the following: "I am a person who can't pay attention very well," "I have difficulty learning," " Something is wrong with me," "I must not be that smart," and "I need to be medicated."

Labels are important from a medical standpoint. They give a foundation for treatment options. But even in that field, a label such as *cancer* can wreck havoc with an individual just as in the field of psychology *schizoid* can do a number on someone already in distress. Labels are helpful to the clinician but should either be withheld or carefully couched on behalf of the client. Remember, talking in terms of *problems* implies solutions.

Now, regarding stress, let's simplify. Stress, which is generated by one or more fears, lack of management skills, plus a host of negative self concepts and beliefs, causes a person to feel out of control to some degree. This internal agitation interferes with the ability to focus. In other words, stress diverts attention. Lack of attention logically impedes learning. That is a universal truism. Finally, can you imagine a person who has no internal fears, no nervousness, a person who is calm and laid back and who time manages well, can you imagine that person not being able to pay attention except perhaps under the circumstance of momentary distraction?

As we have seen, fear produces anger. People use anger as a way to discharge stress, so issues of anger often get tangled up with stress. They may, for instance, feel stressed by the subconscious fear of winding up alone. They discharge that stress by fighting with their spouse, which actually increases the odds that they will wind up alone.

WHAT IS STRESS MANAGEMENT?

Stress management simply means getting back in control. Core Healing does this in two ways—by eliminating the negative self concepts and beliefs that generate the higher levels of stress, and by teaching practical life skills to help people cope with the day-to-day realities of their lives. Mindful meditation, as a life skill is very helpful. Setting priorities and wise time management are essential.

In our society, we tend to be overextended. We are over scheduled, and have too much on our plates. We are often in debt, and don't always have a plan to change that. We may not have good relational tools. We have more wants than time to achieve them all. We don't get enough sleep.

Young people don't get a manual that shows them how to manage their dreams, their relationships, their finances, their "to do's," their children, their scheduling, their housekeeping, or their own sanity. Very few of us are prepared to manage our lives. We are in desperate need of strategies and tactics for living, and skills for coping with the predicaments in which we find ourselves.

Stress Management is both a psychological issue and a practical issue. As we work on removing clients' subconscious negatives such as worrier, perfectionist, "I'm a disorganized person," "I am the one who must handle it all," etc., we also work on life management issues. The four most common predicaments people find themselves in that assures life in the speed lane with inadequate time for restful sleep are: less income and savings than are needed; too many wants that have been allowed to exceed the means; a job that works them like slaves; more children than time of day to provide routine, quality attention; not enough time to wind down wisely at the end of a day and have a minimum of the at least eight hours of sleep now known to be required for healthy functioning. The trapped feelings resulting from feeling "in over one's head" can be overwhelming. Something as simple as creating a schedule for oneself becomes essential. It is a way to begin getting into the solution which helps to manage anxiety. The absolute priority must be self care oriented, and most especially, starting one's schedule with adequate time for wind down and sleep. One by one, practical solutions are discussed pertaining to each dilemma in which the person finds himself. Often recommended to a couple is getting a good financial planner, a house keeper if affordable, a smaller house, and any other ideas that seem appropriate.

Everything is directed toward getting them back in control of their lives.

STRESS MANAGEMENT STRATEGIES

The absence of adequate life skills can exacerbate, as well as result from, our negative self concepts and beliefs. For instance, Nancy was taught as a child not to be selfish. Her self concept of "I don't deserve to put myself first" resulted in putting everything and everybody else first, to the point that she felt completely out of control of her own life.

Nancy didn't have the life skills to distinguish between "positive" selfish—taking good care of herself—and the "negative" selfish of running roughshod over people. We want to be there for people, but we need to be there for ourselves first. It's a little like what flight attendants tell us about the oxygen masks on a plane: "Put on your own mask first, then help others."

People who are stressed out are often already in the whirlpool—even drowning. They need immediate help with practical planning, almost always in the areas of time and money management. For instance, the pregnant woman who is stressed out about not having the resources to care for her baby needs to sit down with a pencil and paper and figure out how much time and money are involved, whether or not she has that much time and money, and where she will get it if she doesn't have it. Ideally, these are before, not after, pregnancy issues.

In addition to deleting and replacing negative self concepts and beliefs, Stress Management in Core Healing also includes:
- Time management
- Money management
- Information gathering
- Informed prioritization
- Self discipline
- Problem solving
- Responsibility (the ability to respond appropriately to situations)

- Anger resolution
- Critical thinking: distinguishing between needs and wants, for example

This understanding of the difference between "needs" and "wants" is crucial (Maslow, 1968). Many people let the circumstances of their lives drift out of control because they do not, or cannot, make this distinction. They may *want* an expensive new car, but not *need* it and not recognize that the unnecessary financial burden it creates can build stress for them and for their family.

Here are some examples of the difference between "needs" and "wants."

NEEDS	WANTS
Nourishing food	Food variety/quantity/gourmet
Safe shelter appropriate to climate	More than 1800 square feet for a family of four
8-10 hour of sleep	Getting along on less sleep
Financial security (in the form of adequate savings)	Acquiring more than we can afford in order to impress others or feed a false sense of esteem
Balance among work, play, exercise, quiet time, time with family, time with nature/God, acts of love, learning and personal growth activities, and vacations	Expensive destination holidays, buying expensive cars and clothing to impress or fill emptiness. Millions of dollars with which to control others as a way to assuage one's fears of not being lovable and/or inferiorit

When we pursue our "wants" at the expense of our "needs," the inevitable result is stress. When we combine lack of all the above life management skills with core fears and negative self concepts and beliefs, then we become stress machines.

COMMON NEGATIVE SELF CONCEPTS AND BELIEFS

Some of the most common core fears associated with stress are winding up alone, being abandoned, being unlovable, not being good enough, and being worthless, inconsequential, inferior, or stupid.

Why do people get in over their heads? We have seen that it can be a simple lack of practical skills, but it can also be a form of self abandonment—often exacerbated by self concepts such as "I don't know how to manage money," "I'm just a spender, not a saver," or "I'm too stupid to figure this thing out."

Difficulty sleeping often suggests that self abandonment is at issue, as does the dynamic of women feeling as if they are not good mothers unless everybody else comes first, and they come last. Norah was only sleeping four hours a night. She had "back burnered," or abandoned, herself in favor of handling her husband and children's needs. The result was that she became more stressed, slept less, abandoned herself more, and so forth into a downward spiral that resulted in acute anxiety and depression. After we dealt with her misguided and subconscious belief that she deserved to be abandoned, Norah was led to incorporate the wisdom in Rabbi Hillel's words: "If I am not for myself, then who will be?... And if not now, when?"

Other negative self concepts and beliefs associated with stress include:
- "I have to allow the 'authority' people in my life to be in control of my decisions."
- "Everyone else is more important than I am."
- "My happiness does not count."
- "I am a spendthrift."
- "I abandon myself (which includes being obese, broke, addicted, or whatever dis-ease is dictated by other constellations of beliefs)."
- "I don't know how to get organized."
- "I fly by the seat of my pants."
- "I am supposed to be a parent in order to have worth, or to be accepted."
- "I have to have 'X' number of children."
- "I don't pay attention to time."
- "Five hours sleep is all a person should need."
- "I don't know how to create a time nor money budget, let alone live within

one."
- "I don't have time to think about what is important in life."
- "I am a natural worrier."
- "I have to do everything just right."
- "I am too stupid to figure things out."
- "I am not responsible."
- "I am scared to make up my own mind."
- "I am a worry wart."
- "I have to get everything done yesterday."
- "I can do it all...work, raise kids, be a wife, clean house, etc."
- "I am always late."
- "I am lazy."
- "I can't think straight."
- "I think the world is a dangerous place."

CASE STUDY: Judy

"I'm a basket case!" Judy told me. She was 32 and expecting her third child under six. Her husband Todd made a decent salary, and they had decided she should stay home and take care of the kids until they were all in school. But they hadn't exactly planned on this third child, and for the past year they had spent more each month than he had earned and eaten into their small savings.

"I don't know what we're going to do, and some days I don't know where to turn next, so I wind up sobbing on the couch. I know that's not good for the kids—but I'm at the end of my rope. They need my attention, Todd needs my attention, my mother broke her hip last year, and I'm afraid we're going to wind up living in the car." She had given up her morning jogs with a neighbor who also had children. She had stopped going to her book club, and rarely socialized except for Todd's work related gatherings.

The "life management" part of Judy's stress management program was pretty obvious. She needed a working schedule that included time for herself, jogging, the book club, and spending time with friends. She probably needed some help with the kids, which she might be able to combine with spending time with her mother if her mother came over to help out three afternoons a week.

But none of that would work unless Judy also dealt with the negative self concepts and beliefs that had contributed to her getting out of control. Judy had come from a wealthy family. Her mother had a nanny, a cook, and several other servants. At a family Thanksgiving gathering the year she was five, Judy overheard two of her aunts gossiping about her mother.

"She's spoiled rotten!" one said.

"She can't do anything on her own, she's just a parasite!" the other replied.

Judy came away from that incident with several subconscious beliefs, among them:
- "People hate women who get help with their families."
- "You should do everything yourself."
- "Good mothers do everything."

When she found herself in a predicament that additionally produced financial uncertainty, an unplanned child, and the panic she felt watching their savings go down instead of up, the stress began to snowball.

We uncovered, deleted, and replaced these negatives so that Judy could proceed with the practical part of her Stress Management Program. She and Todd needed to make and live by a new budget that included the new baby. If they couldn't do that on their own, they needed to meet with a financial planner. They needed a clear sense that, if they did what they planned, everything would be okay.

Stress is a given in our society, and it is easily exacerbated by negative self concepts and beliefs. Core Healing clears those up, so that we can move forward into practical solutions for coping and thriving.

Chapter 10
SUBSTANCE ABUSE

Substance abuse is about self medicating. Ironically, it is also a way people attempt to control something not in their control. Substance abuse is learned by observation, as a way to salve emotional and physical pain, and as an inappropriate way to deal with fear and anger. In the most general of terms, substance abuse is about managing anxiety and depression plus the pain inherent in such predicament.

Substances like food, alcohol or drugs may be used to numb pain, even if only temporarily, and give people a minimal sense of control or escape in the short term. But sooner rather than later, abusing substances makes them feel even more out of control. Substance abuse, in part, is an attempt to *cope*—an attempt that almost always backfires and makes matters worse.

The information in this chapter applies both to prescription drugs and non-prescribed substances. These include alcohol, nicotine, sleeping pills, pain killers, anxiolytics, food, marijuana, cocaine, crack, amphetamines, etc.

GETTING RID OF LABELS

We have seen how labels such as "depressed" or "anxious" can reinforce people's negative self concepts and actually perpetuate these conditions. Where substance abuse is concerned, it is even more important to avoid labels.

The words "addict" and "alcoholic" are thrown around very freely today. In my opinion, using these words is not helpful. It invites people to think of themselves as "addicts" or "alcoholics," which makes it easier for them to adopt behaviors that they associate with those labels—not the least of which is to continue abusing their substance of choice (alcoholic behavior), struggling daily not to succumb (the conduct of an addict) and expecting to relapse (what addicts tend to do).

Alcoholics Anonymous, Overeaters Anonymous, Narcotics Anonymous, and other 12-step programs have good intentions when they invite people to introduce themselves as "an alcoholic" or "an addict." They want to get people out of denial about their unhealthy dependencies. My problem with this practice is that the self concepts of "I'm an addict" or "I'm an alcoholic" get reinforced each time they introduce themselves. It creates more of a problem than that which already exists. Being "addicted" implies that, at best, it will be difficult to stop—but more likely, a day by day struggle. I don't want Core Healing to be difficult, so I ask people who come for substance abuse to stop referring to themselves as "addicts." Instead, I urge them to think of themselves as people with a problem. We all have problems, and problems can be solved—sometimes quite easily. We've all heard people say, "I used to drink (or smoke, or use drugs), but I don't do that anymore." So, rather than introducing themselves as "an alcoholic," it might be better to say something like, "My name is Susie and I have a problem with alcohol." That sounds far easier to resolve.

By the way, people with a severe drinking problem, created it when they made the decision to drink specifically for the purpose of getting drunk, blotto, out of it, gone. This is a different decision than that of one who drinks to take the edge off when socializing. This person's self concept is that of social drinker. A "drunk" is more likely dealing with significant emotional pain, anxiety, depression and the intense fears and the underlying fears and angers that produced it. A "social drinker" is dealing with one degree or another of anxiety. More precisely, the social drinker is dealing with the fear of feeling safe around people with whom they do not feel entirely secure.

THE ROOTS OF SUBSTANCE ABUSE

Substance abuse has many roots. Some of the most common are:

Shyness

Shyness is a huge contributor to substance abuse—especially the substances of alcohol and marijuana, which are dis-inhibitors. The self concept "I am shy" is usually imprinted in childhood. We saw in Chapter 3 that, as animal beings, we are naturally wary of strangers and of those who are bigger than we are. We also saw that when children are introduced to their parents' friends, they often "shy away" and try to hide. They are told, "Now don't be shy!" Then the parent turns to her friend and compounds the problem with, "Oh, you have to excuse Bobby, he's shy." Rather than being complimented on his appropriate caution, Bobby now has the self concept that he is a shy person—and that shyness is bad, possibly even shameful.

Shyness is terribly uncomfortable and can result in isolation. Bobby will do whatever he can to assuage the resulting discomfort of loneliness as well as the conflicting fear of being alone. If he fails to overcome his shyness, he may become more reclusive and introverted. When he is older, he may use alcohol and/or marijuana. These drugs reduce the inhibition to socialize. Smokers have often begun smoking to "be one of the gang." Similarly, those who feel like dregs will do street drugs to at least have the company of whatever others will associate with them. Hard core street drug users are so out of it much of the time they don't particularly care who they hang out with.

Fundamentally, human beings are not loners. Loners are made, not born. It is our animal nature to hang together whether we talk about flocks, droves, packs, schools or bands of brothers and sisters. We want to socialize and be part of a group. Bobby may use drugs, or alcohol, to overcome his shyness. What substance(s) he chooses depends on the degree of his fear, his other negative self concepts and beliefs as well as subsequent reinforcing events.

Clients who come to Core Healing for substance abuse often say things like, "I do well with socializing and having fun when I'm under the influence—but when I'm not, I revert back to that other person, the shy person." How this statement can be interpreted is that they in fact have the social skills they need to have fun when relating to others. They couldn't exhibit such skills if they didn't have them even under the influence. They just need to get rid of the negative self concept of being "shy," so they can live in that truth. That way, the conscious mind's desire and decision to socialize comfortably and be more outgoing will not be impeded by the negative self concept "shy" plus any other related ones found in its constellation. Constellation deletion results in no 'need' for the drug of choice, at least not for that purpose.

Rebellious Reactions

Rebellious reactive decisions are also a frequent factor in substance abuse. Most parents tell their children they can't use substances like alcohol, nicotine and drugs. Or, they can't have dessert if they misbehave. One of the most common reactions is, "Oh yeah? Watch me!" Or "I'm old enough to do what I want!" Or "You can't make me!" Almost as night follows day, kids reach for what their parents forbid—in many cases, just to prove that they can.

This is partly an attempt to get control, something children and teens want desperately. "I'm in control of my own life. I can do what I want!" Of course, abusing substances almost always involves a loss of control.

Learned Dependence

We have noted frequently that when parents do everything for their children, the children never learn to take care of themselves. This learned dependence is an enormous factor in substance abuse.

Kids grow up with the self concept, "I can't make it on my own." When they realize that the time is soon coming when they have to be out on their own, they become terrified. Quite often, they use substances to numb the fear of having to be responsible for their own life. Naturally, this makes the controlling parents feel as if they have lost control. In one extreme case, Frank started drinking and smoking pot at sixteen as a reaction to his overly controlling parents. He was just experimenting, but when his father caught him smoking pot, he took Frank to a mental institution to be treated for addiction. This was serious overkill. Now Frank had the self concept that he was an "addict" and also, since he was in a mental institution, that he was "crazy."

Frank's case is dramatic, but the fear that they can't make it on their own is epidemic among people who abuse substances. At about fourteen or fifteen, they start getting anxious. They know that when they get to be about eighteen, they will be expected to take care of themselves. Live independently. They will either get a job, or go off to college. This prospect can fill youngsters with terror. They are acutely aware that they don't know how to handle their money, their relationships, their schedule, their work, their dishes, their house, or even their laundry. Getting a job may seem overwhelming. They think, "I don't have a clue how to get along in life. I don't know how to earn a real living. I don't have an education. I don't even like school. What am I going to do?"

The closer they get to the time that they're out on their own, the higher their anxiety. They may turn to alcohol first. If that doesn't alleviate the anxiety, and if pot doesn't do it, they graduate to something stronger. Long before they are actually on their own, they have been through a progression of substances that has escalated along with their fears.

It is a predictable cycle. The learned helplessness creates anxiety and often depression. Substances are an attempt to medicate the depression and the anxiety. The higher the anxiety and depression, either bingeing or stronger drugs are used. Bingeing is symptomatic of stark terror. What doesn't *change* is their dependence on something outside themselves. That began with their parents, and continued with the substances. Becoming dependent on a substance is a logical extension of being raised to see oneself as a dependent person...dependent on someone or something for survival.

Eventually, they do leave home—but often they continue to medicate their anxiety and depression with substances well into adulthood. So long as the feeling that they aren't up to being in charge of themselves remains, they continue to use external factors—people, circumstances, or substances—to control them.

This need to look outside themselves for control can exist even when children have been well instructed in the practical matters of life. While such skills are helpful, parents who insist on controlling every aspect of the child's behavior—when and how they do everything, down to the smallest detail—and enforce their authority with anger or shame, then children develop the habit of looking outside themselves for control and direction. They may be great at balancing their checkbook, but not know how to assert themselves in a relationship. When they are always looking outside themselves for authority and control, it may be only a matter of time before they reach for substances to at least feel a modicum of their being in control, a paradoxical conundrum.

When people get some small measure of temporary control and relief, they can start believing that the substance is the reason they are able to manage or cope. They may even believe that if some is good, more must be better. They begin a process of collecting constellations of reinforcing beliefs about the value of the substance. Then they ultimately feel betrayed—and the substance itself becomes a problem, too. Their modicum of control evaporates. Their fears escalate.

Numbing

People who are in emotional and/or physical pain are in a state of dis-ease. The pain may be felt as mild to intense. Its duration may be intermittent or constant. It would be great if an occasional aspirin was all that folks needed. Sadly, that is not the case.

Physicians have been putting forth a mighty effort to deal with pain management, s have psychotherapists, physical therapists, nurses, and all those dedicated to easing pain and suffering in the world. Be that as it may, the problem of pain, emotional and physical, is raging out of control. Millions of pills ingested, millions of gallons of alcohol consumed, millions of cigarettes smoked, millions of hours spent in one form of therapy or another isn't stemming the tide. Hurting children and adults are turning to street drugs, in frantic search of alleviation. Numbing, the escape from pain, is their goal.

Obviously, numbing can not be the goal unless we are dealing with intractable pain. *Curing the source of the pain is the goal*—it is the goal of Core Healing.

COMMON NEGATIVE SELF CONCEPTS AND BELIEFS

Substance abuse often suggests intense, primal fears, as in scared to death. Such intense fear involves abandonment, not feeling lovable, being alone, an aversion to being responsible for oneself, feeling helpless, being shy, feeling worthless, and not worthy of existence. These fears also impel people toward the social aspect of addiction. Even though they may believe that they deserve to be abandoned, they nevertheless want other people in their lives because loneliness can certainly be painful. They are seeking a peer group, and often they believe that the only group who won't reject them are other "addicts." These are sometimes the only people with whom they feel relatively comfortable and accepted. For many, this is one factor for the adherence to AA, Overeaters Anonymous, or Narcotics Anonymous meetings.

Eventually, people hit bottom. At that point, they either kill themselves or change direction—usually by going to AA or some other recovery group. Often, these groups also teach practical and emotional skills that people need in order to cope with life. It is said that when someone starts abusing drugs or alcohol, their emotional maturity stops at that exact point. With the support of groups who understand this dynamic, people can learn to be responsible for themselves, build self esteem, and cope both with their emotions and with the practical aspects of their lives.

In addition to the fears mentioned above, some common negative self concepts and beliefs of people who abuse substances are:
- "I'm scared."
- "I am a rebel."

- "I am shy."
- "I have to be perfect."
- "I need to look 'macho' (by drinking a case of beer)."
- "I'm not good enough."
- "I need excitement because I feel so dead inside." (Danger provides excitement. Street drugs, for example, is a good way to find danger.)
- "I'm angry, and I don't know why."
- "I am empty and purposeless."
- "I have no defenses against a dangerous world."
- "I can't stop spinning my wheels."
- "I can't take care of myself."
- "I'm afraid of success because I'll pRobably lose it."
- "Nobody will ever love me. I'll die alone."
- "I won't fulfill my purpose in life."
- "I need a substance (alcohol, drugs, food) to release pent up emotion."
- "I deserve to be abandoned."
- "I'm unlovable."
- "I'm stupid."
- "I'm a nervous person."
- "I'm inadequate."
- "I have to point out other people's flaws so mine won't be so obvious."
- "I am unmotivated and sad, so any progress I make is slow."
- "I don't know how to be responsible for, or in control of, myself."

The beauty of Core Healing is that it can go directly to the heart of the problem. I ask people who come to deal with substance abuse, "If you did *not* have a headache, would you go to the medicine cabinet and take a couple of aspirin?" Of course, they wouldn't. Then I ask, "So if you didn't have the anxiety or depression, and if you had a great job and were earning a good living, and felt able to handle life independently, would you need that substance anymore?" Not likely! They wouldn't be in physical or emotional pain, and could go forward into their lives with a sense of self-reliance and the self satisfaction that comes from feelings of competence.

CASE STUDY: Stan

Stan was an inveterate smoker. He had tried to quit tens of times, and failed. Finally, he heard of Core Healing. In addition to being "a diehard," he told me that cigarettes were a way to keep his anger in check and his weight down. They were also a way to take "mini-breaks" and, he admitted sheepishly, to keep others at a distance. "Smoking cigarettes fills something up in me that nothing else does," he said.

I have heard many smokers label themselves "diehards." This self-definition, of course, compounds the problem. With that idea in place, they have to act out that definition. Quitting has to be extraordinarily *hard*, maybe so hard they will *die*! Or, they may believe that is the way they are meant to die...the hard way. But Stan was willing to entertain the possibility that he could quit easily if he could identify and delete the negative self concepts and beliefs that had led to his smoking.

Under hypnosis, Stan returned to the most critical, most relevant memory related to smoking. The memory that emerged was in his mother's womb. He felt himself suspended in the amniotic fluid, and became aware that his mother was agitated. She was telling her husband, his father, that she was pregnant. The father became enraged and said, "How dare you get pregnant!" In the next instant, he savagely kicked his wife's belly. Even though Stan was suspended in and protected by the amniotic fluid, he felt the turbulence and was terrified. He felt *as if he shouldn't exist*. (Being kicked to death by someone you are dependent upon would certainly be a hard way to die.) This self concept was imprinted into his subconscious as a felt sense in the midst of the trauma.

We also uncovered a constellation of reinforcing beliefs, including:
- "I am terrified of those on whom I am dependent."
- "I'm a nervous person."
- "I don't trust others not to hurt me."
- "I'm unworthy, not good enough."
- "At times, I feel like an outcast."
- "I am weak/defenseless."
- "I deserve to be abandoned."

Smokers often have these same negative self concepts and beliefs. In addition, as they grow up, they observe older smokers. Their subconscious absorbs the belief that their kind of uneasiness and discomfort can be managed with cigarettes - just as it seems to for those they observe. While quite the opposite is true, it appears to be the case. Nicotine is actually a stimulant, not a relaxant. Nicotine constricts the blood vessels, which means the heart has to pump harder. But the subconscious is so powerful that it actually makes smoking *seem* like it is relaxing. Moreover, smoking seems relaxing because they are briefly distracted from the stress of the moment during the time it takes to light up and smoke the cigarette.

After deleting Stan's negatives, we placed in his subconscious the "personality of a non-smoker," which included a sense of belonging here, being meant to exist as well as being optimistic, outgoing, forgiving of self, and easygoing. Because we were dealing with his subconscious, these ideas were simply accepted. His conscious, logical mind had been saying for years, "Yes, of course! It makes perfect sense to quit. I don't want to be a smoker." But until his subconscious got on board and the negatives were replaced with positives, he could never quit.

Stan said at the end of our sessions, "I can't believe I gave all that power to a piece of paper with dried leaves rolled up in it."

Even after he stopped smoking, Stan found that his hands were restless. They kept fidgeting, and he had trouble holding them still. I asked him what he had liked doing with his hands over the course of his life, other than smoking. He said, "You know, when I was a little boy, I used to like to whittle." He was then in his 60's. "As a matter of fact, I know a whittling class I could go to. Whittling would be more fun to do with my hands than smoking."

Once people are free from the negative self concepts and beliefs that drove them to the substance, they have a lot more energy to be creative and use their lives more fulfillingly.

Chapter 11
EATING DISORDERS:
Obesity, Anorexia, Bulimia

We all know that eating disorders are epidemic and agonizing, and that they cause health and mental health problems that cost billions of dollars a year.

What many people don't know is why they are so *persistent*. The reason is that most medical and psychological models treat only the symptoms, not the source. Even when people begin eating normally for awhile, and either gain as would an anorexic or lose the appropriate amount of weight as would someone obese, they are likely to return to their old ways until the underlying negative self concepts and beliefs are discovered, deleted, and replaced.

Eating disorders have at their core *primal fear*—as in scared to death, as in *freaking out scared to death*. As animal beings, we are wired for self preservation. Trigger the fear of being abandoned which in childhood could lead quite literally to death and the whole of a person, both mind and body, comes reactively into play for self preservation.

When developed to the hilt, the following negative self concepts and beliefs, lead to the degree of fear necessary to foster a full blown eating disorder: Unlovable as is, imperfect, I must be perfect as in thin, even flawless, I am fat, I am ugly, I deserve to be abandoned, I love to eat especially junk food, am scared to be alone, I am not supposed to be the one in control of my life, food is a balm, I am not attractive nor pretty enough, and/or food is a weapon are common.

The three eating disorders that result depending on the exact composition of the relevant constellation are obesity, bulimia, and anorexia.

OBESITY

Fat can be deadly. I refer to obesity as "death by fork." The death is not just from heart disease, kidney failure, or diabetes. It can be a death of love, a death of joy, a death of mobility, and a death of self respect.

Negative self concepts and beliefs control our relationship with food in many ways. Most obese people want to be thinner in their conscious minds, but the subconscious is choosing "fat." We talked in Chapter 1 about people who lose hundreds of pounds after gastric bypass surgery, only to regain it eventually because they have not dealt with the subconscious negatives that were behind the weight gain. We will never solve an eating disorder with a pill or surgery. There is no medical magic bullet. There must be attendant changes in the belief system of the individual subconsciously. Conceivably, that could happen during the trauma of pre and post gastric by-pass surgery.

When diets *do* work, it's because the pros of being trim are at least temporarily in the majority. If diets work, and the weight loss is permanent, that means there is a preponderance of positive self concepts and beliefs in support of that trim image of selfhood. If the weight returns, that means the negatives *outweigh* the positives. Pun intended, the scale's balance is tipped.

When diets fail, sooner or later, additional negative self concepts and beliefs are developed. A few examples are, "I am a person who can't keep my weight down" or "I'd rather eat what I like than feel so deprived." So the next time a diet is attempted, it becomes more difficult with each failure. Future efforts become more easily defeated because they are supported by the additional negatives. The more cycles of weight loss and weight gain, the sooner the failure and the less the success, the less willpower acknowledged, the more helpless we feel. "I'm powerless over food" then joins the constellation of other negatives. The more negatives accumulated, the more failure becomes assured.

Sometimes obese people just throw in the towel and give up trying to lose weight. That is when the real trouble begins. The fatter we become, the less mobile we are. The less mobile we are, the lower our muscle mass becomes. The lower our muscle mass, the more slowly our metabolism functions. We gain more weight with less food. Fear increases, leading to more food consumption, and we feel more and more and more out of control.

Common Negative Self Concepts and Beliefs

For millions of people, obesity is the strategy of choice for counteracting loneliness, for self punishment, for suicide, for dealing with feelings of not being lovable, using fat as a fortress to keep from being hurt, fulfilling their self concept of being fat, and on the list goes.

Obesity as a strategy is sad. Fat is not beautiful. The reality is that fat just produces more and more pain emotionally and physically as the years go by.

The three most common underlying emotions among obese people are fear, rage, and pain. Some of the most common negative self concepts and beliefs leading to obesity are:
- "I deserve to be abandoned."
- "I deserve to be punished."
- "I'm disgusting."
- "I cannot control my eating."
- "I'm unlovable."
- "Sweets are a treat, and eating them makes me feel good as well as loved."
- "I am a fat person."
- "I need to absorb the pain of those around me."
- "I have to belong to the Clean Plate Club."
- "I am genetically predisposed to obesity."
- "Food is the only companion I trust or want to give me comfort."

The following are some specific negative self concepts and beliefs I've heard from obese clients over the years:
- "My Thanksgiving was horribly ruined, so I'll enjoy feasting every day."
- "Now that my children have been born and because I don't care about sex, I'll get myself fat and unattractive to keep my husband uninterested."
- "I'll make sure I never get raped again. I'll get so fat no man will want—or be able—to get near me."
- "By being fat, I become invisible. People don't want to look at fat people."
- "I need someone to supervise my weight loss, just as my mother did when I was a boy."
- "I need to hide my genitalia." (As a girl, this client was thrown out of the house naked by her angry mother. Even though she pounded on the door and begged her mother to let her in, her mother was in no hurry to do so. The child was not just angry, she was enraged. Moreover, she felt ashamed of her genital region being exposed. As an adult, her obesity served two purposes. One was to keep her secure from being exposed. Hanging abdominal, fat engorged skin covered her genital region. The other was a

matter of vengeance. Her grossness was specifically geared to make her mother feel like a "gross failure.")
- "By becoming fat, I won't be tempted to be sexy or seductive. That way, I will honor my marriage vows."

Comfort Food

"Comfort food" is food that has a loving association. On a subconscious level, people have learned to associate particular foods with love, family, loved ones, even to the point that they develop additional self concepts such as "I love Fig Newton cookies," or "I love pasta," or "I love bacon grease to season my green beans." These are redolent of secure times.

Comfort food can be about soothing the loss of a loved one. In other words, the specific "comfort food" brings close either the person who is loved and who has passed on or the love that was felt around that person. For instance, I used to eat a full meal, and then after dinner sit down and have cookies and milk. I wasn't even hungry, but when I was a little girl my mom would always make my favorite cookies for me. It was a way of saying, "I love you, because I'm taking time to make your favorite cookies." So when I wanted to call back that comfort after she passed on, I ate cookies. One client's father loved Fig Newton cookies. She was close to her dad, so Fig Newtons became her comfort food when she needed him "near."

"Genetic Predisposition": A Different Perspective

Many obese clients have said to me, "I have a genetic predisposition to being heavy. Everybody in my family is fat." When looking at the person, obviously it looks like they may in fact be structurally large. Be that as it may, if they were not abusing food, what size would they actually be, as opposed to the size they are? Moreover, consider the client's language. "Everybody in my family is fat." Fat results from bad eating habits. That is a learned behavior from generation to generation. It is not a genetic issue. Structurally, being big boned, or, where fat deposits itself is a genetic issue. We must teach clients the difference.

In working with obese clients, I have learned a great deal. Another important learning is that each overweight person is precisely the amount of overweight they want to be, subconsciously. There is a "fat point" *unless* they have "thrown in the towel" for whatever the reason. If that has happened, then the grossly obese individual is intent on death by fork, and/or absolute dependency as a result of immobility, living like the "filthy animal" they have been name called as a child or teen (personal hygiene becomes a major problem) and fulfill an utter sense that they deserve to be humiliated even degraded, and, finally of course, that they deserve to be abandoned. With these types of horrific self concepts in play, their weight gain knows no bounds.

With individuals who have a set point and are steady at a certain number of pounds overweight, one of the things I do while they are in hypnosis is say, "So, you weigh seventy-five pounds more than you want to weigh (or whatever the amount is for that individual). Let's take those 75 pounds and ask how many of them are attributable to which negative self concepts and beliefs." Many of them are stunned at first, but while hypnotized, almost every client can easily ascribe a certain number of pounds to each particular negative self concept or belief—and do so with remarkable clarity. They might say, "Well, fifteen are due to anger mismanagement. And maybe another fifteen to my belief that it's all genetic." That's thirty. Another twenty five pounds are there to keep myself from having a sexual relationship that might turn out to be painful. That's fifty-five. We keep going until we have accounted for all seventy-five pounds. Then in the Healing Phase, all these explored reasons are turned around into better self concepts to fortify the person in their resolve to be seventy-five pounds less.

ANOREXIA

The symptoms of anorexia are self-starvation or minimal eating. Anorexics see themselves as "too fat." When they look into a mirror, they see a fat person—even when someone standing next to them might see "skeletal." When you actually show them that their bones are sticking out, their subconscious blocks that reality to assist in the implementation of their negative self concepts and beliefs. In some cases that negative is "I might as well be dead because I am too fat to be perfectly beautiful and therefore lovable."

And "too fat" is not thin, and therefore not loveable. Young girls who become anorexic or bulimic have usually been taught to believe, and very often by their fathers, that they have to be thin, even to the point of perfectly thin, in order to attract a man. Frantic fears of not being attractive enough, not lovable enough, or not sexy enough fester in the subconscious, demanding that these girls be "perfect," which they often interpret as "having no body fat." They become literally "scared to death" of winding up alone because they are unattractive, imperfect, and thus being an embarrassment to their parents.

This well of terror is deepened if they are counseled unsuccessfully, and they begin a cycle of compulsive behavior. They feel doomed to being abandoned and unloved if they are not "perfectly thin," so getting and staying thin become the focus of their lives. But they can never be thin enough to achieve their goal of not being abandoned—because *the fear of being abandoned or unloved came before the attempts to be thin.* Trying to lose weight without first dealing with those negatives is like the tail wagging the dog.

The Body of Boy

What drives the conduct of some anorexics is wanting the body of a boy. This has nothing to do with sexual orientation. They have simply observed, and their subconscious has accepted, that they are not as desirable with the body of a girl, and by extension that of a or woman.

Generally, this self concept is imprinted just before, or at the onset of, puberty. One client's father used to roughhouse with her and her brother. But as she started heading into puberty, the father stopped roughhousing with her and just played with her brother. In her immaturity, she came to the conclusion, "Having the body of a boy will get Daddy to play with me again." She was feeling abandoned by her father. The dad was pRobably just aware that she was developing into a young lady, felt a little uncomfortable, and was trying to observe some propriety. But what he was actually thinking had nothing to do with what she interpreted and imprinted. Her subconscious interpreted, "Being a boy is better. I must look like one."

If you are a girl who wants the body of a boy, you learn to starve yourself so that you don't have breasts and so that you develop amenorrhea (absence of periods). That way, you are more like a boy.

Not all anorexics want the bodies of boys. Some simply believe, "I'm fat and I can't be thin enough, and I won't be loved unless I'm thin." This proceeds into, "And if I'm not loved, I'll be alone, lonely, and a disappointment to my family." Some go further, into "Even God won't love me." From that point, there is only the abyss.

Common Negative Self Concepts and Beliefs

Some of the most common negative self concepts and beliefs that generate anorexia are:
- "I deserve to be abandoned."
- "I'm unlovable."
- "I'm too fat."
- "I can never be thin enough."
- "I'll be alone and lonely."
- "I need a man to take care of me, and I'll never find one because I'm so fat."
- "My parents will be disappointed in me unless I get married and have a family."
- "I'm not desirable as I am."
- "I'm so fat and out of control, I might as well be dead."

BULIMIA

Bulimia is the mismanagement of food through a cycle of binging and purging. Symptoms can include weight loss, ruptured esophagus, balding, teeth falling out, malnutrition, and electrolyte imbalance. Those who are bulimic are afraid they will be unloved, and therefore isolated, if they are "too fat." They will not be worthy of a man in their life.

Anorexics and bulimics have similar underlying fears, but their strategies are different. Bulimics often enjoy eating. They really like food and want to "have their cake and eat it, too." I had a client whose husband always bought her chocolate, which she loved. She wanted to enjoy the candy, and also to please him, but she was terrified of getting fat—so she would eat the whole box and then throw it up.

Terrified of not being thin, or thin enough, people who suffer from bulimia often starve themselves during the day (a metaphor for a fear of love starvation), or eat quite sparingly and judiciously. Come night time, they fortify themselves at a nearby supermarket with the binge du jour. It might be a package of cookies, a cake, three bags of potato chips, or whatever. Frantic stuffing at night manages the dis-ease of feeling deprived and/or starved by the time they get home. It allows the individual to indulge their comfort food(s) upon which they depend for the implementation of such a self concept as "chocolate makes me feel better." Obviously, by the time they are getting home they are not feeling too great, hence *chocolate* cookies. Eating them all stuffs down one set of their sources of terror. Purging then happens as a strategy to deal with a whole other set of their fears such as "I dare not get fat". They have been taught that if they are fat no guy will want to marry them, no loving nourishment, no family of their own, which then means winding up all alone and into a primal type fear of dying alone.

Anorexia and bulimia can overlap. Suppose someone is anorexic not because they want a boy's body, but simply because they have bought into the idea that they are too fat and can't be thin enough. They might become bulimic as a strategy to be "thin enough." Bulimics are more likely than anorexics to approximate a normal weight. Anorexics often get so thin that it's life-threatening, succumbing to the negative belief, "I might as well be dead because I am too fat."

Common Negative Self Concepts and Beliefs

The bulimic's negative self concepts and beliefs are similar to the anorexic's. The intensity of these beliefs, and the nature of the constellations around them, determine whether someone becomes an anorexic or a bulimic or rotating between both predicaments. These negatives include:
- "I deserve to be abandoned."
- "I am too fat, and therefore undesirable and unlovable."
- "I'm not good enough the way I am."
- "I'll be alone and lonely the rest of my life."
- "I don't deserve to exist as I am."
- "I have to look 'perfect.'"

CASE STUDY: Anna

My client Anna tells her story better than I could:

I was in my early thirties when I went to see Dr. Glasser, and weighed 325 pounds. I had gone up and down all my life, and had weighed as much as 480. I'd lost hundreds of pounds many times, but it always came back. I just couldn't do that again. I needed something beyond will power, so that I could keep it off.

I was at rock bottom, and scared. I was either going to kill myself with diabetes or some terrible heart problem, or I was finally going to do something that brought success. I wanted this to be the last time I lost that weight, and I was willing to try anything and give 100%. I think that was part of why I succeeded.

I was an emotional eater. I swung back and forth between salt and sugar. It was a bag of chips, to a box of chocolate, and back to a bag of chips. I never ate in a healthy way, and I was definitely a closet eater. You didn't see me eat anything, yet I still weighed almost 500 pounds. I knew what I should be eating; I just put a whole different set of food in my mouth.

I had done a lot of traditional psychotherapy, using the conscious mind to discuss various issues, but I was never able to resolve anything at the core level. It would just get me by for the time being, but I kept going back to the same way of eating.

Along with the food and weight issues, I had relationship issues. I always put myself last. I tried to please everybody, went above and beyond the call of duty for the people in my life, and put everybody else's needs before my own—family, friends, and business associates.

I liked hypnosis. It was very gentle, very pleasant. I went back and discovered some things that happened when I was two or three years old that were very powerful. I realized that I'd adopted subconscious beliefs back then that were still running my life today. Some of them were:

- *"I'm not smart."*
- *"I'm not capable."*
- *"I can't be successful at anything I try."*
- *"If I'm thin, I'll be exposed."*
- *"People will expect more of me if I'm thin."*
- *"If I don't do what people expect of me, I won't be loved."*

It was a recipe for exactly what was going on with my body and my relationships. I had this incredible release, this "Aha!" when I saw it. We went back through each emotion, each negative belief, to the bottom of each of those rabbit holes—that's what I call them—until it was completely empty and I'd blown off all the emotional charge. Then we came back up, replacing each of those false, negative beliefs. When it was over, they just didn't exist anymore.

That was two years ago, and my life is very different now. I have literally shrunk to less than three quarters of my size in a year and a half. I now weigh 195. At 5'9, I look like a normal person. I did that because I believe in myself and want to be healthy. And it has held, where it never did before.

<u>My motto is: Ice cream doesn't taste as good as thin feels.</u>

I say to myself, "Okay, we're only going to eat things that are good for our body, because that's what our body deserves! It doesn't deserve to be on a sugar high, and then on a sugar low, and then on a salt high, and then on a salt low." I eat well not because I "have to," but because I want to honor myself. I eat three full meals, may indulge in a piece of chocolate here and there at a party, but I am satisfied at the end of the day. I do step aeRobics and salsa dancing, and I love it.

My relationships and friendships are very different now. The people who are my friends now really like and respect me. It's a mutual exchange, whereas previously it was all about me trying to please them. These are rich, lifetime friendships with people who are on the same long-term goal path that I am.

I'm much more aware of my own emotions than I ever was before. I always held things in. I never cried in front of my parents, for example. I never told them that I loved them. I'm much more open now to telling my siblings and my parents that I love them and more open in showing emotion.

I had always been a very tough, hard businesswoman who didn't show her feelings. That's how all my friends from Iowa knew me. But the people I've met in recent years, here in Florida, see me as this warm, sensitive, loving person. I had a big 40th birthday party with both groups there. They were sitting around the table, taking turns saying things about their friendships with me, and the people from the Midwest said, "When I met her, I thought, 'I want to get on the good side of this person!'" They were a little scared of me! The Florida people said, "This is the most gentle, giving person we've ever met!" It was night and day.

All of us were amazed!

But the greatest gifts have been freedom and self esteem. I had been my own biggest obstacle in life—and I'm out of my own way now. I have the freedom to think what I want to think, and not be afraid of life, and try things that I never would have tried before—knowing that some of them will work out, and others won't, and that's okay. I like myself.

I healed from the inside out, and that feels great!

Chapter 12
PURPOSELESSNESS

Purposelessness is a sense that we really don't know what life is about, what our own value is, or what we should be doing. It is a subtle, but pervasive, condition—and an important factor in many physical and psychological dis-eases.

Purposelessness is characterized by confused or absent values, and a sense that our lives have little or no meaning—or else that there is meaning out there somewhere, but we don't have access to it. The religious, family, and societal values that used to define our purpose in life have for many become blurred, at best. People without a strong spiritual base can easily find themselves drifting.

We want to know:
- Does what I do really matter?
- How important is it?
- Do I make any difference that counts?

These questions suggest a more fundamental question: *Is what I'm doing good enough?* This, of course, reflects the core fear, "I'm not good enough" or the negative self concept "I have nothing of value to offer; I am worthless." For the most part, we do not have clear, lasting, in depth answers to these questions—and this sense of purposelessness affects our relationships, physical health, emotions, spirituality, and behavior.

WHAT DOES PURPOSELESS LOOK LIKE?

Vital people feel that what they are doing serves a larger purpose and contributes to life. They are energized by their work and relationships, and know that what they are doing means something to others, to the world, and to themselves. They are able to love freely, and to thrive.

When this sense of meaning is absent, energy flags. Love becomes difficult and complicated. A vague malaise begins to creep in, a sense of not being valuable or valued. "I'm not good enough" starts gathering constellations of other negative self concepts and beliefs.

People whose primary dis-ease is purposelessness rarely come in saying,

"I don't have a sense of purpose in life." Purposelessness is usually *beneath* their presenting issue, which is often depression, anxiety, substance abuse, or a physical problem.

Again, we have the chicken and the egg. Are they depressed because they lack purpose, or do they feel as if they lack purpose because they are depressed? In Core Healing, it doesn't matter. Many of the same constellations can give rise to either depression or purposelessness. Since the aim of Core Healing is to root out and replace all negative self concepts and beliefs, it is more efficient when we begin with what the client views as their most pressing of problems first.

ROOTS OF PURPOSELESSNESS

Purposeless usually begins early on, in the home, and is often a function of values empty of altruism and low expectations of the child. The classic example is little girls being raised to believe that their purpose is to get married, have children, and serve their families. If that is their single purpose, or even their primary purpose, what happens if they get divorced, if they can't have children, or if their children or spouse die? What happens when the kids grow up and leave home? Their whole identity is gone, everything that told them who they were and gave their lives meaning and value. What now? Maybe there are grandchildren, but maybe not. Maybe they have a lot of interaction with the grandkids, but maybe not. Where do they go from here? What is life about now?

Purposelessness can also grow out of having been taught that one specific thing is of value—and not following that particular path. Kevin's father always wanted him to be a doctor. He was raised to believe that value and purpose came from being a professional who served others in this particular way. Partly as a negative reactive decision and partly because he loved music, Kevin became the keyboard man in a rock band. The band was actually very successful, but Kevin wound up getting involved in drugs. Under hypnosis, he identified the belief that "I haven't done anything of value with my life." He had actually done quite a lot; it just wasn't the one thing that his father had identified as valuable.

Prevention

One of the jobs of a parent or teacher is to notice and acknowledge their children's strengths, and to make their children feel like winners. We all have unique talents and abilities, and kids get off to a better start when they are recognized for being smart in school, or good at sports, or great at drawing, or particularly kind to people, or diligent about whatever they do, or capable of bringing joy with their laugh, or whatever it is that they do well. Children who grow up in this kind of environment often have a subtle, built-in purpose. They know they are good at something, and that their particular "something" has value. Their parents gave them this message early on, and it got imprinted on their subconscious. Likely and subsequently is was positively reinforced. Acknowledgment of a child's true strengths as well as their thoughtful development lays a foundation for their helpful use. Placing a child on a pedestal with undue praise or for shallow effort, on the other hand, fosters Narcissism.

Teachers also need to seek out and praise the skills, talents, and accomplishments of their students. Who is terrific at math? Who is good at reading? Who knows how to support other people on the team? Who is always generous about helping others? Who hit the home run on Saturday? Who has a knack for science? The more people are praised for what they do well, the more their attention and energy go in that direction. They develop more positive self concepts, and come away with a higher sense of purpose. Like parents, teachers are in the perfect position to create winners. When children know they have gifts, they can hone and actualize them. This gives their lives confidence and the recognition of what they have that can be used with purpose.

Often, kids' unique talents and abilities are revealed by what *interests* them. "I'm interested in music" can translate into "I'm good at music." "I like math" can translate into "I'm good at math." "I like dinosaurs" might mean "I like biology, or history, or zoology."

If parents and teachers stay alert to these kinds of messages, they can teach based on competency. Many schools are already doing this. It's a very simple system. If my competency is music, I might learn to read and write by reading about music and musicians and writing short pieces based on what I read. Interest- and talent-based learning results not only in *more* learning, but in fewer discipline problems and in children with more purpose in life. By the same token, focusing on what children are *not* doing well reinforces negative self concepts. Focusing on their improvements, serves improving.

Finally, we must inspire children into a purposeful life as I was inspired as but one example by the motto from my high school: The North Shore Country Day School in Winnetka, Illinois. The motto is *Live and Serve*. In Judaism, it is a dedication to *mitvot*, doing good deeds. In Christianity, the meek, the gentle and the kind, shall inherit the earth as they love their neighbors as they love themselves. (Loving *self* wisely and well would be an important subject to teach.) In Buddhism, there is a dedication to compassion. How then can a life not be lived purposefully and well when one is committed to service (to others) in the form of good deeds conducted by a person who is gentle, kind and compassionate with their neighbors,

COMMON NEGATIVE SELF CONCEPTS AND BELIEFS

Purposelessness can grow out of just about any constellation of negative self concepts and beliefs. A few that often put in an appearance are:
- "I'll never amount to anything."
- "I'm not good enough."
- "I'm worthless."
- "I'm unimportant."
- "I'm inferior."
- "I'm no good."
- "I'm going to hell."
- "Even God doesn't love me because I've never done any good with my life."
- "I'm stupid."
- "I can't do anything right."
- "I never do well. I might as well give up."
- "Nothing means anything. Why should I even try?"
- "I always fail, and I'm tired of it."
- "I'm a loser."

Often, people's sense of self-worth is so diminished that they can't conceive of what they might have to give to anybody else. The following are some of the negative self concepts and beliefs discovered by one client for whom purposelessness was a key ingredient of his depression and eating disorder.
- "I am a bad person."
- "I don't deserve respect from others."

- "I deserve to be abandoned."
- "I am afraid of dying."
- "Food takes away pain."
- "I don't deserve to be heard (as in children should be seen, not heard)."
- "I can't get full enough—of love, of food."
- "I deserve to be abused."
- "I am not grown up enough."
- "I can't be alone. It's too painful."

CASE STUDY: Evan

Evan was thirty-four years old, the Public Information Director for a large nonprofit organization. He came to Core Healing for depression. He was depressed, but it seemed to me that there was something else going on as well. When he did his "Why?" questions, we found among them:
- Why do I have trouble getting out of bed in the morning?
- Why do I just want to zone out in front of TV when I get home from work?
- Why haven't I done more with my education and talents?
- Why can't I connect with people on a deep level?
- Why do I sometimes feel relieved when I get sick and can stay home from work?
- Why do I not have any faith in God, or in what might come after death?
- Why do I worry so much?
- Why don't I get excited about things?

Under hypnosis, Evan recalled a time when he was four. During nap time, he had crept into his mother's room and was happily eating away at a pound box of chocolates she had on her night stand when Evan appeared in the doorway out of nowhere. Feeling exposed and likely ashamed of herself, Evan's mother shouted at him."What are you doing?" Evan felt a flush of shame over his whole body. "You little pig she screamed (a projection), you'll never amount to anything (the feelings she was assuaging with the chocolates)." Startled, frightened, these negatives flew directly into his subconscious, lodged there firmly, and began collecting constellations of supportive negative self concepts and beliefs. (Not surprisingly, Evan had weight issues as well. "I'm a little pig," with all the shame and terror that surrounded it, became a magnet for like beliefs.)

An extraordinary number of people have Evan's subconscious negative self concept, "I'll never amount to anything." This particular one almost guarantees a sense of purposelessness. Even when people are raised in homes with strong religious and ethical beliefs, as Evan was, there is very little hope that they can live up to those standards or values. After all, they will never amount to anything. Even if they know the "right" things to do, they won't be able to do them. So, why bother? It seems as if there is nothing of value within to share.

After deleting that self concept, and all the similar ones that had gathered around it over thirty years, we replaced it with beliefs that built self esteem, such as:

- "I am a person with unique talents and abilities." (And these strengths were specifically identified.)
- "I choose to be of service to people."
- "I contribute in my work, and with my family."
- "What I do is important."
- "I deserve to be excited about life."
- "I deserve to acknowledge and reward myself."
- "I am a skilled and generous communicator."
- "There are things I have done that in fact, contribute to people and make their lives better."
- "I deserve to enjoy life."

Six months later, Evan told me that he and his wife were off to Nepal for a trip that had always been their dream vacation. He was enjoying his job and colleagues, and had started to write a book he never felt he could do. He wanted the first one to be to help children based on what he had learned. Finally, he reported that he woke up each morning with a sense of well-being, knowing that he had a reason to be alive, an important job to do, and many people who loved and appreciated him.

Chapter 13
UNHEALTHY ATTRACTIONS

There are various forms of unhealthy attractions. One type, sex addictions, is about a figurative type of impotence, as in powerlessness. The fear of a loss of power and/or feelings of being out of control are incredibly intolerable for these folks. We only need power when we are afraid we do not have it or are afraid of what might become of us if we lose it. This type of unhealthy attraction, based on a demand for prodigious sexual involvement, is primarily an anxiety management issue. Moreover, it can be reflected upon as another type of substance abuse issue as in Chapter 10. In this case, the substance abused is the bodies of the participants.

Another type of unhealthy attraction derives in significant part from a sense of entitlement. Commonly accepted boundaries that we as human beings have established are waived. One such boundary is marriage. Entitlement suggests the idea that one's pleasure supercedes abiding by the law. The idea that marriage is a legal, and as is often invoked a God's boundary, is dismissed or ignored. Potential consequences for such boundary crossing may fleetingly come to mind but are dismissed in the heat of seduction. Hedonistic entitlement combined with potent subconscious beliefs of the negative types described below make for unhappiness at the least and the potential for combustibility at its worst.

WHAT DO UNHEALTHY ATTRACTIONS LOOK LIKE?

A woman comes in for therapy. She presents her problem in these words, "My husband is cold and uncaring. I go to him for a little affection, and he pushes me away. Am feeling so isolated in my own home." And then she might add, "This is my third marriage, and, it seems like I keep marrying the same man. They have different names but the same M.O. They all treat me indifferently. How can that happen when while we were dating they were so warm and attentive?"

We all know people who have a pattern of attracting certain kinds of partners. Some may have a high turnover rate in relationships—but even though their partners have different faces and different bodies, they are really the same person, over and over again.

It's almost as if people *need* that certain kind of relationship, no matter how much they protest that they want something different. A man might choose women who cheat, or flirt, or spend too much money, or let themselves go, or focus only on the kids, or nag, or lose interest in sex, or whatever it is that makes him crazy. The woman might choose men who are cold and uncaring, or bullying, or ignore her and the kids, or have affairs, or beat her up, or are momma's boys, or turn out to be gay, or whatever makes *her* crazy.

Unhealthy attractions very often occur when the negatives that we observed and absorbed in childhood dictate the way we think people are supposed to be, what roles each are to play, how couples are meant to interrelate.

THE ROOTS OF UNHEALTHY ATTRACTIONS

Children are sponges, and much impacting data prior to the age of three goes directly into the subconscious. The development of logic, which is left brain activity, is just beginning to develop. How well ones logic develops depends on the environment of the child. If it is almost exclusively faith based, reason and logic are not as embraced and consequently not well developed nor applied. A wholesome balance between faith and reason is critical.

We observe our parents' behavior—and get the message that *that* is how men, or women, or spouses, or people in authority, or partners behave! If Daddy didn't hug the little girl, she may well become attracted to men who aren't affectionate. If Mom always berated the little boy, he might find women who do the same. We may wonder why we choose men who are physically or emotionally absent, or women who have a short fuse. The answer is simple. Fathers are people who are *gone*. Mothers are people who *scream*. As we grow up, we generally recreate our first families with great precision.

We may complain, "Why aren't you *there* for me?" The reason is that we picked someone who *wouldn't* be there. We've all heard the phrase, "He knows just how to press my buttons!" Of course, he does. That's why he was chosen! And it's a double whammy, because this *dynamic can cross genders*. The woman can find herself with men who recreate dynamics she experienced with her mother, and the man can "marry" his dad! It gets even more complicated, because we were chosen by our partners based on what went on in *their* families. Sometimes, it can feel as if we're living inside a pinball machine. To make matters worse, most of us are unaware of the subconscious negative self concepts and beliefs that are driving this bus.

The dynamic of recreating our original families allows for positive imprinting as well, but here we are concerned with unhealthy attractions. More often than not, we get attracted to the worst in our parents, the things we say we would most like to change about them, instead of to the best.

HOW IT WORKS

Imagine being two, three, four, five, or six years old and looking up into a world of grownups. They may be there for you, or they may not. Imagine the visceral fear of watching these big people screaming and shouting, slamming doors and perhaps even being physically violent with one another. There is no place to go, except maybe under the blanket or into the closet.

When we are very young, as mentioned earlier, we do not have sophisticated critical faculties. We simply absorb what we witness in our homes. As far as we are concerned, that's how life is. Our parents or care givers are our most immediate influences, and our most powerful ones. We absorb many of the self concepts and beliefs we see in them—whether they engage in a loud war with one another, wage more discreet offensives, are illogical in their thinking, simply keep one another at arm's length, misuse drugs, act anxious, physically or verbally abuse one another, stay married or get divorced. These self concepts and beliefs about husband, wife, marriage strongly affect our choices about significant others later in life—whether we adopt the same self concepts and beliefs our parents had, or whether we rebel and make "never again" reactive decisions against what we witnessed.

Generally, we take on, we replicate their dis-eases. We assume their emotions and the thought patterns that produced them, their behaviors such as worrying, their stressors, their attitudes about life and about God.

In Chapter 6, I described one exercise we do in Core Healing to root out these negative self concepts and beliefs. I ask clients under hypnosis to imagine themselves around the age of six, looking up at their mother. I ask them to imagine that they have one wish, and only one wish, about one way their mother would have been different. Ben might say, "I wish she had hugged me more." Then we start "peeling down."

Therapist: What difference would that have made?

Ben: I would have liked myself better.

Therapist: And what difference would it have made if you'd liked yourself better?

Ben: I would have had more friends, and chosen women who liked me better.

Therapist: And if you'd done that, what difference would it have made in your life?

Ben: I wouldn't have chosen women who nagged and berated me.

Therapist: And what difference would that have made?

Ben: I might have had a happy marriage, and children.

In the Healing Phase, we can now work with the self concept, "I don't deserve a woman in my life who is affectionate with me." Also, this type of dialogue is used constructively to remove any resentments with his mother. In doing that, it is imprinted on his subconscious an adult/adult, forgiving interaction with her. An additional goal is that in the future he won't slide into similar child/parent relationships with women, especially any that might remind him of his mother from a negative perspective. Then we repeat this process with Ben's father and other significant people in his life, discovering more negatives.

When we have those parental inputs, we bring in all the "exes," that haven't worked out and have them stand between the parents. If Ben wishes his mother had hugged him more, or his father had paid more attention to him, I ask, "What about Sally? Was she like your mother or your father in those ways?" Very likely, Sally will resemble one or both of his parents in the ways he wished they were different—and so will all the other women who "haven't worked out," because Ben's template for a wife is someone who ignores and/or mistreats him. One at a time, we examine the relationships until they are complete.

With Vicky, it might be that "husbands" or "men" are people who are "gone," or who hit their wives, or who disappear into the newspaper or television all evening. That is her template. It's what she learned from the earliest significant man in her life, her father, and it is *what she believes is the way it is supposed to be.* Based on such subconscious imprints, she will seek out men like this and usually fall for them until those negative self concepts and beliefs are erased and replaced.

In the Healing Phase, we replace the negatives with positive self concepts so that people are attracted to those who have the best qualities in their parents, plus the qualities to which they want to be attracted.

COMMON NEGATIVE SELF CONCEPTS AND BELIEFS

Here is how negative self concepts and beliefs get put in place. Abby, 5, and her brother Ned, 4, see their father beat up their mother. Abby is horrified and very afraid that Mommy might get killed. If Mommy were to get killed, Abby would be alone and wouldn't survive. After all, daddy goes to work and never plays with her. In a state of fear, this whole scene gets photographed by the subconscious. The trauma witnessed is imprinted along with the emotion of fear and the negative self concepts and beliefs and any reactive decisions.

Later, with Ned watching, the negatives are compounded when Mommy comes to her and says, "It was my fault, honey. I knew your daddy doesn't like me to talk to him when he first gets home from work." The mother is trying to soothe Abby, but she is actually teaching her to believe:

- "It is okay to be hit by your husband if you did something he told you not to do."
- "Whenever someone hits you, it is your own fault."
- "Husbands give orders that are to be obeyed. If you don't obey, it is okay if they punish you."
- "This is how a wife acts—obsequious and servile, the placating peace maker."
- "This is what a marriage is like."

Ned picks up these beliefs:
- "Wives are to do what you tell them. If they don't, you beat them up to punish them."
- "Men are the bosses in a relationship."
- "Women are there to do what you tell them to."
- "This is what marriage is like."

If Abby doesn't erase and replace these beliefs, she will be the perfect, albeit unhealthy, match for a boy who grew up with the same beliefs as her brother did. Together, they would recreate their idea of "home," "family," and "marriage."

That is how negative history repeats itself. Abby's "Why?" questions might look like this:

- Why do I fear being alone, and yet at times prefer it?
- Why can't I find happiness?
- Why do I have such a hard time saying "No?"
- Why do I take on too much?
- Why am I married to someone who doesn't love me?
- Why do I allow things to get so bad between my husband and myself?
- Why do I put everyone's happiness before my own?
- Why can't I leave my husband, even though he abuses me?
- Why does it seem everyone else's life is more important than my own?
- Why do I get so nauseous when my family argues?
- Why do I doubt people's motives when they are being nice to me?
- Why did I marry a man who never saw the good in me even when we dated?
- Why do I have to always play the peacekeeper role?

Ned's "Why?" questions might be:

- Why do I lose my temper with my wife over the least little thing?
- Why did I marry someone I don't respect?
- Why do I seem to marry the same kind of woman every time?
- Why can't I make my wife do what she is supposed to do, just by telling her once?
- Why do I like sex better with prostitutes?
- Why do I spend my spare time looking at porn on my computer?

Some negative self concepts and beliefs that commonly compel people to choose unhealthy relationships are:

- "I'm not lovable."
- "I don't deserve to be given time or attention."
- "I can't take care of myself."
- "I deserve to be abandoned by the man (woman) in my life."
- "I need someone to depend on to control me."

In the Healing Phase, of course, we would replace these negatives with

positives like:
- "I deserve someone who will be there for me."
- "I am attracted to people who know how to balance work and personal commitments."
- "I am lovable and attractive."
- "I deserve someone who treats me with respect and kindness."
- "I can take constructive control of my own life."

CASE STUDY: Susan

Susan is a New York attorney. We worked on a variety of issues over the years, including being attracted to emotionally unavailable men. She was forty-five when we did this work. Before then, she had experienced other therapies. In her own words...

> *The other therapies just didn't hit the real issue. I was married to my first husband at the time, and he was extremely distant and emotionally unavailable. We'd talk with the therapist, but without hypnosis, all my defenses stayed pretty much intact and we never got to the central issues that would change my attitudes and behavior. I had always dated men who abandoned me, and I was even choosing as friends and colleagues people who would abandon me.*
>
> *Under hypnosis, we went back to the original incident that started this whole thing. I was five years old and sitting on the steps of our house, listening to my mother and grandmother having this enormous, knock down drag out fight. These two women were very important to me when I was five. My mother and I had a very touchy relationship. I was much closer to my grandmother, and had lived with her when I was very young. Now I was back living with my mother. That afternoon, with all the yelling and screaming, I was absolutely terrified and panicked. Here was my mother, who I wasn't that close to but with whom I had to live now, in a battle with my grandmother, whom I loved.*
>
> *In my conscious, adult memory of this event, I just*

remembered being "angry and disappointed." My adult mind had remembered it in a way that was distant from the full range of feelings I had at the time. But under hypnosis, my subconscious was called upon to make the full awareness of the memory surface. The experience, as my subconscious recorded it, offered great clarity as to the actual magnitude of the fear this event caused me. I reactively decided "I have to find someone who never does this!!! Someone who will never scream or holler!" So I always chose men who would never go toe to toe with me, who completely backed off from any kind of conflict, <u>and who therefore were emotionally unavailable</u>.

My first husband filled the bill perfectly. He was safe and stable and dependable. I liked that a lot, because my past had not been safe. But he was not fun. He was intellectually smart, but he was stubborn and had no "give," no humor.

Under hypnosis, I got down to about fifteen incidents that all reinforced that original incident with my mother and grandmother. In the Healing Phase, we looked at how I could go back and help that five year old process the information differently. My adult self could help her see that, "These are adults handling a situation very badly. It really has nothing to do with me. They still love me, they still care for me, and my life will go on unchanged even though they're acting this way."

Of course, when I was five, that kind of thinking would have been a big stretch. But under hypnosis, I could actually go back, be in that experience, and handle it the new way. <u>And as far as my subconscious was concerned, after Core Healing, that new way was now my guiding way.</u> The old negatives were just completely gone! It literally changed the perception of the memory, changed the decision I made not to engage in relationships that might have any kind of inflammation around them.

Instead, I had the new belief, "You can have a disagreement with somebody without putting up your dukes. You can even have an argument without it becoming the core pain of your life." I didn't have to hold on for dear life, trying to control everyone and everything around me so that I never had to experience something like that again.

I saw that we always have a choice about how we digest an experience. If you decide to take a different message from the experience, and you do so at the subconscious level, you simply eliminate the bad choice. So once you process the past in a different way from how you processed it back then, <u>you just don't have those negatives anymore</u>. Core Healing is like donating old, outdated clothes. Once they're gone, you don't even notice that they're gone.

My next relationship was with a man who was completely different. He was kind, fun, and emotionally available. We were well matched intellectually, and there was just a flow about us. He was just what we had programmed in the Healing Phase, except we forgot to program for good health. He and I had a wonderful relationship for two years, but then he passed away.

My current husband is wonderful—available, smart, supportive, and playful. I know that if we have a disagreement, it won't be the end of us. I'm not afraid to invest in the relationship, or to have someone close who actually engages with me. I'm more relaxed about my friendships, too, a lot calmer and less uptight. And I'm better by myself than I ever was before. I'm living inside my own system, and it's a very nice place to be.

This kind of healing is like grace. I felt like God "engraced" me. You don't earn or deserve grace; it just comes in. You have to do the legwork, but you can be "engraced" to go on to the next part of your life relieved of that burden. It gives me so much gratitude. I can't think about this work and not be awed and grateful.

I'm a divorce lawyer. I see people all the time who have been in therapy three times a week for twenty years, and they've gotten nowhere. They may get succor and support, but they don't change their lives.

The greatest gift of Core Healing is being close to people—

to love my husband, my son, my friends, and my colleagues. I know now that if there is something negative in my life, I can fix it. Nothing has to stay the way it is, if it gets in your way. Once you have these tools, you know that anything is possible.

Chapter 14
ANGER RESOLUTION

Anger is a natural human reaction, but it does not occur in a vacuum. It erupts in response to feeling that we have been treated unfairly, to feeling demeaned, and/or to feeling frightened or hurt. In this sense, anger is a secondary emotion. The fear, hurt, or feelings of injustice or being demeaned must occur *first*. Anger is simply a reaction to these precipitating, primary emotions.

Additionally, anger can be a conditioned response, a kind of knee jerk reaction. X situation calls for the A response. This cause effect relationship, this pattern of conduct is learned. There are still negative self concepts and beliefs behind it but the anger response was simply called into play based on the 'right' situation. Even though anger in and of itself is a passionate response, nonetheless, it can be dispassionately executed. Wife does or does not do X. Husband whacks her and calmly resumes watching football.

We all get angry from time to time. The question is: What do we do with it? Anger can be expressed appropriately or inappropriately. Appropriate expressions of anger are diplomatic, understanding, compassionate, and focused on creating win/win situations. These modes of expression lead to resolution. To respond this way, we need to be able to see things from the other person's point of view, and to gain whatever skills or knowledge we need to negotiate a resolution.

Inappropriate expressions of anger include passive/aggressive, hurtful, to frighten and thereby control, and/or punitive. As an attempt to control another, exert power over another, it becomes bullying. (Bullies are made, not born.) Bullying, a learned behavior, is generally founded on self concepts such as being weak and inferior, and/or, it is my job to control others for my own purposes, what I want or need is more important than what you want or need, intimidation is a way to control others, I enjoy feeling this kind of power. Anger can also be used to exact retribution demanding the "eye for an eye." Then too anger is used as an attempt to mitigate one's own pain. Sadly, this tactic works when a person has the self concept that causing retaliatory pain makes one feel better. This kind of anger perpetuates the problem - and usually makes it worse. It results in more pain, more isolation, and more anger.

Part of Core Healing involves expressing appropriate, compassionate anger toward members of the client's Cast of Characters, those who caused them grief. At the same time, we are imprinting the kinds of attitudes, conversations, and tools needed to resolve anger in a positive way. A client's belief that ugly anger is acceptable is deleted, and replaced with self concepts of being a forgiving, entirely responsible and compassionate person. Models for constructive anger resolution are given under hypnosis, and people are positioned for success in handling anger more appropriately.

I may even "rehearse" anger resolution during hypnosis. I might, for instance, suggest to the client that he imagine that he is driving down the highway. Suddenly, someone cuts in front of him, scaring him. But now he understands that fear is simply fear, and that he doesn't have to slip into the secondary response—anger. Rather than yelling, honking, and gesturing to the other driver in a way that would undoubtedly escalate the situation, he can react in a way that is more appropriate (and safer!) because he can observe the situation clearly. The other driver, who is likely harried and sleep-deprived, may be angry himself, or simply careless, or perhaps distracted. The client calms down from the fear, and lets the danger pass. He sees that he handled a difficult situation well, and gives thanks for being safe.

Core Healing gives people the means to find healthy resolution to anger, rather than slipping into reactions that are fiery, hurtful, controlling, irresponsible, passive/aggressive, "tit for tat," or condescending.

HOW ANGER WORKS

Many people who have a problem with anger are painfully aware of it. They have been unable to control their temper, and have gotten in trouble. Other people come to Core Healing with other difficulties, and discover that anger is beneath their presenting issue. Obesity is a good example of this. The more severely obese the person, the more likely they are to be dealing with rage. Still others mask their anger with passive/aggressive behavior—acting nice, or at least rational, on the outside while finding ways to "stick it" to the other person. Consciously or subconsciously, they believe that it is simply too dangerous to express their anger directly.

Anger is a learned behavior. Whatever we see our parents and other role models do with anger, that becomes our model. We might grow up in a home where people scream and throw things. Or where fights are loud, but not physically abusive. Or where nobody ever speaks about being angry, but you can cut the tension with a knife. In the latter case, expressing anger becomes something to be avoided at all costs. People with severe problems expressing anger are often afraid that if they ever let themselves get angry, they might wind up killing someone.

Anger is all around us, not only in the news of the world, but in the supermarket, in families, and on the road. Road rage is a form of anger that has gotten a lot of attention lately. It is epidemic, the result of over scheduled, hurried people carrying around overloads of fear. Their out of control anger is a release valve. They are already worried when they get in the car to go to work. How will they pay their bills? Can they sell their house? Can they keep their job or marriage? Their mother is in a nursing home. This "worry reverie" is in full bloom when some kid going ninety miles per hour on a motorcycle zooms past them loudly, scaring them so badly they jump. This spikes their stress quotient. The reaction is rage, an explosion of anger.

Road rage is a spewing out of all the repressed energy contained in our swirling, seemingly irresolvable fears. In this case, it was triggered by the terrifying noise from a motorcycle. Our screaming and swearing, in situations like this, are attempts to feel in control when we actually feel quite powerless. We can't catch the kid on the motorcycle and vent personally, so we become "tough."

The "On/Off" Switch

What many people do not realize is that a flaring temper is, in part, a matter of choice. We have an "on/off" switch for anger, at least in the first few seconds that we realize that we are angry. We can flip that switch to "off" in a nanosecond. Or, we can let it rip. If we don't flip it right away, we lose control of the switch based on the instantaneous decision to let a person have it. In that brief window of opportunity, we can decide to let our anger roar, or to deal with it like a lamb. It is not a macho issue. It is about civility and compassion. To deal with anger differently means we have to become different.

Handling anger "differently" can be positive or negative. We may not be yelling at the top of our lungs, but that doesn't necessarily mean we are dealing with our anger in positive ways. "Quietly" doesn't necessarily mean "constructively."

A destructive form of quiet anger might be passive/aggressive behavior—like accidentally on purpose spilling a cup of hot coffee on a co-worker, for example. A positive alternative might be conversation, using the language of conciliation.

Many children grow up with the anger switch pretty much in the "on" position—largely because that is what their parents model. It would never occur to them that they could flip the switch to "off." Their anger is like a cocked pistol, and any stimuli can set off the reflex to fire.

The "on/off" switch is the first practical thing I teach people with anger issues.

ROOTS OF ANGER MISMANAGEMENT

Anger mismanagement, the expression of rage to hurt or control others, requires that we endorse certain negative values. These include:

- Punishment is good.
- Meanness is acceptable.
- Hurting others alleviates my pain.
- Hitting back twice as hard is a matter of self defense.
- An "eye for an eye" is a valid reaction to being hurt.
- It's okay to be thoughtless, inconsiderate, or uncaring.
- How I feel is more important than how you feel.
- It is important to exercise power at all costs.

These are the values of despots, who generally harbor feelings of inferiority, unlovability, and a terror of failure. This leads to a sense of entitlement, grandiosity, and hubris. Anger is how they cope with fear and a sense that they are secretly unimportant or worthless.

To manage and resolve anger constructively, we must endorse very different values that include:

- Dignity and diplomacy
- Fair play
- A desire to seek solutions
- Compassion
- Kindness, gentleness, and loving our neighbors as ourselves
- The unconditional love of self

To manage anger effectively, we need three things:
1. *Knowledge of how anger occurs in its various forms, and that it has an "on/off" switch.*
2. *Elimination of negative self concepts and beliefs that foster the mismanagement of anger* replaced by the values inherent in peaceful resolution.
3. *A positive/compassionate model for handling the primary emotions that precede anger as well as how to manage anger itself,* so that we are free to seek fair resolution.

COMMON NEGATIVE SELF CONCEPTS AND BELIEFS

Anger mismanagement comes at a high price, as in death and destruction. It is the latter result that has caused people to seek therapy with me. One man came to Core Healing not because his anger had gotten him in legal difficulties, but because he was afraid of losing his family. They were simply fed up with his frequent and inappropriate anger outbursts. He looked very tough on the outside, but his greatest, and quite common, fear was "dying alone and unloved." His "Why?" questions included:
- Why, if I am not listened to, do I get violent?
- Why do I always feel guilty?
- Why do I feel like I am unacceptable to God?
- Why do I feel like God has cursed me?
- Why do I never forgive?
- Why do I feel that no one cares about me?
- Why am I so offended when other people speak badly of me?
- Why am I frightened by the evil-doers in this world?
- Why is there something inside of me fighting change?
- Why do I get furious instantly?
- Why do I always look for the negative?
- Why do I cop out on being responsible?
- Why am I jealous?

The following are his negative self concepts and beliefs. They are a good example of how our negatives can contradict one another, and how fear forms

the basis for anger:
- "I'm a black sheep."
- "I'm weak, worthless, and gutless."
- "I'm too stubborn."
- "I'm neurotic."
- "If I act responsibly, I lose power."
- "I have to control everybody."
- "I'm shy."
- "I don't deserve respect."
- "I deserve to be abandoned."
- "I deserve to be humiliated."
- "I abandon myself."
- "I don't deserve to live."
- "I don't deserve to be loved."
- "Punishment is the way to achieve justice and correction."
- "God hurts and punishes."
- "I deserve to be punished."
- "I need to be controlled."
- "If I 'submit,' I will be insignificant, forgotten, and disappear."
- "Life is not a good thing."
- "I am small."
- "I can't trust myself."
- "I have to be perfect in order to avoid failure."
- "I am terrified of failing."
- "I don't deserve to be taken seriously."

Some common negatives among people who need help to resolve their anger issues are:
- "I can ease my pain by causing you pain."
- "You deserve to be punished."
- "If you hurt me, I hurt you back."
- "An eye for an eye."
- "If you slap me, I feel better if I slap you back."
- "I deserve to be abandoned." (And if you don't abandon me, I'll push you

away with my anger.)
- "I'm unlovable."
- "I deserve to abuse and be abused."
- "I am not responsible for what happens to me. You are to blame."

LEARNING TO RESOLVE ANGER

Everyone knows that, under certain circumstances, it's not appropriate to have a temper tantrum. Once we decide not to "blow our top" publicly, we have another decision. Will we deal with the anger constructively, or subvert it into other behaviors. Crying is one release mode when verbalization or physical demonstration are prohibited. Smoking is a good example of substituting another behavior for that of anger.

Richard told me, "If I'm at work and one of my co-workers makes me furious, I know I'll look like an idiot if I have a full blown temper tantrum at the office. I don't want anyone to see that side of me. So I just say, 'I need to go for a smoke' and leave for awhile."

Leaving the situation momentarily to get away from what is making you angry is a good idea, but smokers take it a step further. They give the cigarette the power to tamp down the anger. They associate anger management with the cigarette—when in fact, it is the *leaving*, not the cigarette, that manages the anger. Also, smoking causes you to inhale. Pulling the smoke into the body literally feels like it is pushing down, even pushing away the anger. It seems like a way to get rid of it. The problem is that the anger, improperly assuaged, is still there.

This is not constructive anger resolution. It is simply anger suppression. That anger will eventually rise to the surface, often when we least expect or want it. If someone trips that trigger, there may be an atomic explosion. The anger has been building and building. When it explodes, it is usually way out of proportion to the situation that finally becomes the detonator.

When I teach adults anger resolution under hypnosis, I teach responsibility for one's predicament and assertiveness in dealing with it. (Many people present for therapy the fear of confrontation.) The situation resolves not when a guy such as Richard stuffs down the anger, but when he calls the co-worker aside and says, "You know, I get antsy when you come and look over my shoulder when I'm working at my computer. I wonder if you would do me a favor, and not look over my shoulder when I'm working. Would you do that?" By making this request, he creates a contract with the person. He is not stuffing annoyance. He is not just saying, "Please stop it!" He is getting a cooperative buy-in, an agreement. Assuming the co-worker agrees, Richard can then say, "Thanks, I appreciate that. It really will help me focus better." He has made a connection, a contract, something they are doing together. He has also created a template for constructive anger management in future interactions. (This scenario presumes of course that Richard's co-worker is a reasonable person. If not the approach would need altering based on the description of the co-worker's style.)

CASE STUDY: Dana

Dana came to me because she was having terrible problems with her son. They had gone to counseling a few years earlier, but "just chatted." She always seemed to be furious with Ethan. Any little thing set her off, and she would scream at him. She could see that he was becoming habitually fearful, and even seemed to cower around her at times. She was also living with a man, Charlie, who relied on her for financial support. That made her angry as well, and once she even attacked him physically.

Under hypnosis, we got to the source of the anger. When she was five years old, a neighbor accused Dana of stealing her four year old son's toy truck. Dana had not stolen the truck, but her mother sided with the neighbor and punished Dana by making her spend an entire day in her room. (Being treated unfairly was the precipitator, and anger the secondary emotion.) She emerged chastened, but furious. However, she didn't want to rock the boat further, and so stuffed down the anger.

The negative self concepts and beliefs imprinted that day included:
- "I deserve to be abandoned by those closest to me."
- "I deserve to be punished, even when it is not my fault."
- "I don't deserve to be believed and respected."
- "I'm not good enough."
- "I could die, because my mother won't protect me."
- "Even if I tell the truth, I'll be punished anyway."
- "The only way to be angry is to hurt/punish someone."

Under hypnosis, Dana was free to experience the anger and was led to assertively tell her mother how betrayed she felt, how angry she was, and how she wanted to be believed and treated with respect. We created a compassionate milieu in which to heal that relationship. Continuing in the healing phase, we brought in her son and husband. She told them what she had seen, and how she had been taking her rage at her mother out on them. Under hypnosis, she reconciled with them, and also forgave herself. This "rehearsal" made it far easier for her to have the actual face to face conversations with them.

Dana no longer has to lash out for reasons she doesn't understand. She can observe her emotions, step outside them for a moment, and inquire about them rather than simply acting on them automatically. She has access to the "on/off" switch. When her son does something to trigger her anger, she can stop, take a breath, and choose how she wants to not simply react but thoughtfully respond. She is in control, and doesn't have to explode or become violent. Nor does she have to stuff down her anger. She can talk with her son and husband, tell them what has upset her, and come to a resolution with them. The result is that she no longer feels weak or victimized by them.

She has a whole new relationship with her mother as well, one based upon respect and on the love they have always felt for one another despite their difficulties. Dana is able to let her mother be as she is, and to communicate honestly when they have differences. She says, "I figure she's not going to be here forever, and I don't want to have any regrets. Life is too short to harbor all kinds of resentments. I still have my days, but I have an attitude of gratitude. I'm grateful for the things I have in my life. Letting go of the anger was a big first step. It's easier now to deal with things that bother me. I know I have a choice. I can get angry about it, or not. Moods come and go, but I don't go down the tunnel with them. I try to put things into perspective."

Dana felt a new spiritual depth as well after Core Healing. She doesn't belong to any particular church, but says, "I'm just more in tune with the world and nature, and the energy that is life. I appreciate what I have rather than getting angry about what life hasn't offered me yet. My way of being spiritual is to try to be good to people. As just one example, I try to say hello to the guy who takes my money at the toll booth, because he's a human being just doing his job."

It's not that Dana never has trying days, but she has imprinted tools that help her to keep from sinking into feeling helpless and lost, and therefore angry.

"This has been a life-saver for me," she says. "My son is eighteen now and we have such a great relationship. He used to be timid and a little afraid of me. I was not someone he wanted to cross. Now if we have a disagreement he'll say, 'Mom, we always figure it out. So let's not discuss it when we're angry with one another. Let's talk about it when we've calmed down, because it always works out.' He's taken my model and made it a whole lot better. I'm now learning from him!"

Chapter 15
PHYSICAL PROBLEMS

We have seen that the subconscious can actually influence what happens in our bodies. I believe that most, if not all, of our physical dis-eases have their roots in subconscious negative self concepts and beliefs. Traditional medicine has long recognized the connection between certain mental states and medical conditions (Rossi, 1993) like high blood pressure, fibromyalgia, migraines, irritable bowel syndrome, heart disease, and even cancer (e.g. Siegel, 1986).

HOW IT WORKS

Our bodies always strive toward normalcy, health, and homeostasis. Illness occurs when something disrupts that normalcy. I believe that fear, painful memory containment, anger harboring, negative self concepts and beliefs, feeling routinely out of control, plus self punishment and self abandonment are our main sources of disruption. They reside within through no fault of the host. Moreover, the particular ways dis-eases manifest—why one person might develop migraines, while another gets high blood pressure—is a function of each person's role models as well as their related subconscious beliefs.

We only keep pain, fear, and anger around for two reasons. Either we haven't yet learned that they can be released, or we are getting some kind of secondary gain from them. We might, for instance, get sick or develop a disabling condition in order to get control of somebody close to us—or to escape some obligation or responsibility, sidestep a confrontation, or avoid disapproval or abandonment. Illness can also be a form of self punishment. It can even result from letting a news broadcast slip into our subconscious when we "space out." For example, we hear a medical report on the radio and think to ourselves, "I bet I'll be the one in four who gets cancer."

Illnesses are often metaphors for what we are feeling or fearing. Anxiety, for instance, can promote high blood pressure that eventually causes us to "blow a gasket."

WHAT CORE HEALING OFFERS

Core Healing's success with physical problems depends not so much on which dis-ease is being treated, or even on its severity, but on the client's belief in the process and his or her willingness to have it work. Be that as it may, working in tandem with the medical community is essential and must be viewed in a way that is not contradictory to the assumptions upon which Core Healing is based. Similarly, the medical community must fully support the power of the mind in fostering healing. Someday, the whole big picture of mind body healing will be adequately researched to begin to make even more definitive assertions. For now, we know of the powerful connection between one's beliefs and one's health as well as our dependence upon the medical establishment for their expertise. It would be foolish not to make it a happy marriage.

Core Healing calls for the release of all damaging emotions stored in the body. I simply suggest to the subconscious that it scan the body to locate any unhealthy emotional deposits and, once they are located, "wash" them clean. We then offer specific healing suggestions appropriate to the client's particular difficulties—enlarged knuckles, irritated joints and stomach lining, other inflammatory problems, heart conditions, cancer, high blood pressure, etc. I often use an image to symbolize this "washing, " perhaps a radiant healing light that washes through every pore and cell, or some other positive visualization that "cleanses" the body of negative emotions.

Under hypnosis, this emptying of negatives becomes easy. Remember, the subconscious, which controls one's physiology, makes no value judgments. It just does as it is told. Unless there are conflicting beliefs (which we would have discovered long before this part of the process), these healing suggestions can be implemented quite simply.

COMMON PHYSICAL PROBLEMS

Can Core Healing work on virtually any physical difficulty? I do not know. I haven't worked on them all. I wish I could say about any problem presented that Core Healing cured them all. What a miracle that would be for us all. However, while I believe the potential is there, we have human factors of which I as the therapist am one and the client the other. We also have some understandable competing beliefs from the medical community. But, if you believe as a result of finding supportive evidence that—thought precedes everything—then Core Healing methods that search for, delete and replace all relevant negative thoughts and ideas with positives could ostensibly cure everything. That of course is broad, but not necessarily, pie in the sky speculation. Landing back on earth, below are some examples that Core Healing has actually been helpful in curing.

High Blood Pressure

Susan had always had 98/60 blood pressure, so low and exemplary that her doctors often thought they had made a mistake and re-took it two or three times. But when her husband became seriously ill, it shot up to 140/95. This was only what they called "borderline bad," but it was extremely high for her. The doctors told her it was just the stress of his illness, and ultimately of his death. Yet a year and a half after he died, Susan's blood pressure was still 140/95. And factor into this situation that Susan is a petite size zero or two, a rigorously healthy eater who works out regularly.

In Core Healing, she realized that the real stress was not so much that her husband had been ill and died, but that she hadn't been able to "fix" him. As a trial lawyer, she was used to winning if she applied enough energy to a situation. She was accustomed to her caring and concern producing a result. She had thought, in her subconscious, that if she worked hard enough, she could heal her husband. "I don't like losing cases—or anything. I like to win, and with him I didn't win," she said.

Obviously, she had lost cases before, but not many. And she had always been able to "contain" her emotions about it. But when she couldn't help her husband, she felt as if something had "slipped." And once it slipped, she was afraid she would be completely out of control. In Core Healing, we worked with her feelings of being out of control, her need to control and fix everything, and her feelings of being completely undone if she could not do so.

That condition had played out for her at various ages and stages of life, so we went back and healed all the younger "Susans" as well. She let go of the fear and anger, and of the idea that either she had to control everything, or she would be completely out of control in her life. *Immediately, her blood pressure dropped to normal.* The doctor told her, "This just doesn't happen. You can't have that high a blood pressure one day, and have it the way it was the next." But she did, because she had released the maladaptive need to control, the fear that she wouldn't be able to do so, and the anger that resulted when inevitably she encountered something she could not control—her husband's death.

"When I could own that I couldn't control it, that I didn't need to control it, and that I could just turn it over to the universe, my blood pressure went back to normal," she said. "I realized it wasn't my responsibility nor in my power to save his life. And it's been normal ever since."

Cancer

We have no idea how much of the information we read, see on television, or hear on radio gets imprinted on our subconscious. A woman came to see me with cancer. I asked her, under hypnosis, to go back to its most critical, most relevant memory. She remembered hearing on the radio that one in four women would get breast cancer in their lifetimes, and thinking that she would be one of them. Within ten years, she had breast cancer.

When we trance out in front of any medium, we are vulnerable to whatever message is being delivered—and once the message has been absorbed in the subconscious, it can manifest in our bodies.

Emphysema

I worked with a man in his early fifties who was an inveterate smoker and had emphysema and heart failure was imminent. He was short and somewhat bowled over. He weighed about 125 pounds, was bloated as a result of poor circulation, and was so weak that he could hardly sit, stand, or even lie down without struggling to breathe.

Under hypnosis, when I asked him to go back to the most critical, the most relevant memory as to why he hadn't quit smoking, even though it was so clear that inhaling nicotine was killing him, it was when his son had died. He felt to blame. (No matter the circumstance, parents, dangerously to themselves, often find some way to blame themselves.) His reactive, subconscious decision in the presence of that trauma was "a life for a life." His instrument for a punishing, agonizing death was the cigarette. Until our work together, his amoral subconscious did an excellent job of complying. During the Healing Phase he was led to a compassionate resolution with himself in a forgiving interchange with his son. (The spirit of a loved one takes form and can exist quite clearly while in the state of hypnosis.) After the session was concluded, his wife took him immediately to the hospital. It was a wonderful team play between the field of psychology and the field of medical science that saved this man's life. Within three months, his symptoms indicative of a failing heart dissipated and his emphysema improved about 70%.

Migraines

Migraine headaches are often a learned behavior, and can carry the secondary gain of giving people a good excuse to say "No" without having to actually say "No." For instance, say a friend invites me to go hiking on Sunday. I may not be all that excited about it, but I agree because I like her and don't want to disappoint. But as Sunday gets closer, I start thinking, "Gee, Sunday is the only day I ever really take off, and now I've told her I'll go hiking. I don't want to go back on my promise, but I really don't want to go."

How do I get out of it? I've learned to be scared of telling the truth. And a headache might not be a good enough excuse, but a migraine is so debilitating that I couldn't possibly go hiking—or do anything, for that matter. If I have a migraine, then I don't have to hike, I don't have to go back on my word, and my friend won't abandon me. In fact, I might even get some attention and sympathy. I don't even have to lie to her, because my subconscious already understands this strategy better than my conscious mind does, and my head has already started to hurt.

Colds are also a great and quite classic way to escape and rest, a legitimate way just to lie down and take some much needed time off.

Irritable Bowel Syndrome

Anxiety affects people in different ways, and in different parts of the body. Some get nauseous. Others get heart palpitations, stiff neck or sore shoulders. Others put the anxiety, fear, anger, or need to be punished into their bowels. The bowel gets hyperactive, so stools are pushed through much more rapidly than normal—to the point that people lose control of their bowels.

I worked with an insurance executive who was constantly on the alert for where the Men's room was because these spasms led to diarrhea. IBS began to govern his life. Under hypnosis, he remembered a time when he was six, and his parents made him recite a short poem he had memorized for the extended family at Christmas. "I have to perform under pressure, or I'll humiliate my parents and they will abandon me" had followed him all the way to the board rooms of Fortune 500 clients. When he released this negative belief and the idea that stomach troubles (in a generalized sense) run in the family, and replaced it with self-acceptance and self-forgiveness, his IBS improved 90%, he enjoyed his work more, and actually performed better!

Birth Trauma

Trauma during the birth process can result in illness later in life, even though the conscious mind does not remember it. These traumas can be "initial sensitizing events." An event in which the newborn is being strangled by the umbilical cord, for example, can become the initial sensitizing event for asthma if it inhibits exhalation, according to Dabney Ewin, M.D., author of Ideomotor Signals for Rapid Hypnoanalysis: A How-to Manual (Charles Thomas Pub Ltd. 2006).

The twisting of a newborn's neck during delivery can be the beginning of migraines. The illness depends not so much on what actually happened, but on what the subconscious did with it based on prior and subsequently developed self concepts and beliefs.

COMMON NEGATIVE SELF CONCEPTS AND BELIEFS

Constellations of negative self concepts and beliefs can result in illness or a debilitating physical condition, just as they do with substance abuse, depression or any other problem. It just depends on the beliefs that compose the constellation(s) as to what problems develop. Different constellations can produce varied conditions in one individual. Some of the most common negatives that produce unhealthy conditions associated with various physical problems are:

- "I am constitutionally weak."
- "Colds and migraines are excellent for getting out of what I can't otherwise assert myself to avoid doing."
- "I am insecure."
- "My stomach is always tied up in knots."
- "My existence makes those I depend on unhappy, so I shouldn't exist." (This can be the case in an unexpected or unwanted pregnancy.) I suspect

that such belief could cause children to commit suicide once they learn a method, such as running out in front of a car.
- "I don't deserve to be heard."
- "I'm afraid to be alone."
- "I deserve to be abandoned."
- "I need to abandon myself for acting like a selfish person (or a loser or burden, or for being born before the parents were married)."
- "I deserve to be punished, and illness is a good way to punish myself."
- "I am not in control of my body; it controls me."
- "I need to be perfect, so people will be happy that I exist."
- "I need to take the whole world on my shoulders."
- "I am a burden."
- "I am not a healthy person."
- "I am selfish because I get what I want."
- "I am not smart enough, and am therefore a lesser person."
- "I am shy, an introvert."
- "Illness distracts me from my fears."
- "I am powerless over others."
- "I am weak-minded."
- "I bloat when I feel a loss of control over my own destiny."
- "I am a bad person."
- "I'm a failure."
- "I am not respected by my father."
- "God will chastise me for not following his teachings."
- "I can't relax."
- "My worth depends on my accomplishment."
- "I can't tell my true feelings."
- "I am sad."
- "I am nervous."

It has been my experience that illness can be traced back to negative self concepts and beliefs. When these negatives are discovered, deleted, and replaced, plus other hypnotherapeutic methods applied, the illness can just disappear. However, it might just get some degree better, or, not get better at all.

The sources for minimal improvement or no improvement can be attributed to the therapist missing something important to therapeutically address, being inept, <u>or</u> the condition is minimally if at all psychogenic.

I predict that within the next fifty years, peoples' beliefs about the efficacy of hypnosis, professionally conducted, will be so entrenched and the methods of hypnotic healing so sophisticated that hypnosis will become a primary tool of physicians as well as psychotherapists. It will supersede medication and surgery in so many instances that hypnosis will be the tool of choice. Moreover, it wouldn't surprise me if the fields of psychology and medicine blend into a powerful whole.

CHAPTER 16

HABIT CONTROL

A habit is a routine way of doing something. Habits can be positive or negative, as William Glasser (no relation) points out in *Positive Addictions* (Harper Row, 1985). Habits are considered "bad" when they interfere with the quality of our lives.

Bad habits are basically systems for mismanaging pain or discomfort. In this chapter, we will look at some of the negative self concepts and beliefs that promote bad habits.

"Habit" needs to be differentiated from "addiction" and "obsession." These conditions are viewed by people as a matter of degree, with "habit" being the mildest form. If "habits" are viewed as easier to take control of than "addictions" or "obsessions"—if only because the label is less threatening and onerous—habits will be easier and the other more difficult to fix. However, when doing hypnotherapy, these distinctions can be explored as a member of the person's constellation. *Definitions* of self concepts construct the individual's behavior. Habits by definition and common perception are less difficult to overcome. "Addictions" and "obsessions" imply by definition, entrenchment, imprisonment, and perpetuity.

Addictions usually involve the misuse of a substance, such as drugs or alcohol. Negative habits generally involve a misuse of self—nail biting, hair twirling, thumb sucking, bed wetting, cuticle biting, eyebrow and hair pulling, rocking back and forth while sitting, etc.

HOW IT WORKS

Habits assuage feelings such as fear, anger, pain, anxiety, discomfort, and feeling out of control. They are often self-comforters, and many people simply switch to another habit when one becomes unacceptable. If parents scream at them every time they suck their thumb, for example, they might use rocking, or hair twirling, or some other habit as a substitute to achieve the same kind of self comfort. Or, the child might become furtive when thumb sucking.

Obviously, solutions rarely come from external criticism or telling people,

"Just quit biting your nails!" Until we relinquish what is behind these habits or some other beliefs surmount the negatives, we don't control them.

Habit control is the ability to choose, consciously and easily, the habits we do or do not want to incorporate into our routines. For example, I like the habits of walking in the morning, reading my newspaper at breakfast, then showering. These habits are adjustable as circumstance require, but I enjoy the routine. It supports my well being, my work, and my enjoyment of life.

Our conscious and subconscious minds must be in harmony in order for us to choose our habits. When there is disharmony, the value we "choose"—exercise, for example—may be abandoned altogether, or chosen only intermittently. Core Healing creates harmony between the conscious and subconscious by eliminating the negative self concepts and beliefs that are behind the habits that seem to control us. That leaves room for, and actually invites, the habits that we prefer and are now free to choose.

HOW WE GET, KEEP, AND FINALLY CONTROL HABITS

Habits are learned behavior. I learned to pull at my cuticle from watching a family member as a child. I absorbed the image and the effect. For me, and for him, it was a pain management system, a way of discharging emotional pain by creating the distraction of physical pain. In my twenties, I had a band-aid on every finger. But as I worked through my negative self concepts and beliefs, I no longer carried that kind of pain—and so I didn't need a way to discharge it.

As children, we observe both bad and good habits, and either accept or reject them in the blink of an eye based on our self concepts and beliefs. Once accepted and adopted, our amoral subconscious reinforces the habit—good or bad—based on the same self concepts and beliefs that initially chose it.

For example, if we adopt the good habit of exercise, we will reinforce it with constellations of beliefs like "I feel better when I exercise," "I focus better throughout the day," and "Exercise gives me energy." There may be competing self concepts and beliefs—"I'm lazy," "I don't like getting up early in the morning," or "I'm an uncoordinated klutz"—that can be triggered and work against the good habit. In the case of exercise, of course, self concepts and beliefs about the body also come into play. We might think, for instance, that we are fat or thin, muscular or mushy, athletic or not, beautiful or unattractive, handsome or ugly, etc.

The swirl of competing and ancillary beliefs can be confusing—until we realize that, by eliminating the negatives, we bring ourselves back to choice. We give ourselves the freedom to choose habits that support us, ridding ourselves of any negative constellations that are contrary to what is in our best interests.

COMMON NEGATIVE SELF CONCEPTS AND BELIEFS

We have noted that many "bad" habits are simply coping styles, ways to discharge and manage discomfort. Some, however, have another purpose as well. They are adopted specifically because they are offensive and keep other people at a distance. This is a tactic used by many smokers. Blowing smoke in and around people who do not smoke is an almost foolproof way to be left alone. It is akin to not bathing or using deodorant. People who use habits to keep others away are likely to have negative self concepts and beliefs that include:

- "I'm an outcast."
- "I am unlovable."
- "I deserved to be abandoned by others."
- "I don't trust people not to hurt or betray me."
- "I should abandon myself."

Occasionally, a habit like nail biting can be dealt with through regular hypnosis, without the work involved in Core Healing. In other words, the therapist can simply hypnotize the client and plant positive suggestions that alleviate the nail biting, without exploring all the person's negative self concepts and beliefs. But I would hate losing the opportunity to "Clean House"—explore for other negatives that might not even have a direct impact on the nail biting—but that are geared to heal the entire person.

There is always more going on that meets they eye. The following are some negatives self concepts and beliefs discovered by one nail biter. Many could manifest as any negative habit.

- "I bite my nails to manage my anger."
- "Expressing anger is a sign of weakness."
- "I have to suppress and internalize anger."
- "I have to work hard for approval."
- "I am sub-standard."
- "I am bad because I didn't do what I was told."

- "I'm afraid of being alone."
- "I am not at peace within myself."
- "No matter how much I achieve, it is never enough."
- "I get picked on." (This was an apt metaphor.)
- "I am defective."
- "I am powerless."
- "I am undesirable."
- "I am not good enough."
- "I have to be perfect."
- "I'm afraid of pain, especially the pain of a failed relationship."
- "Nail biting and cuticle pulling is a way to manage the pain of failure."
- "I'm a loser."
- "I'm a quitter."
- "I need someone in my personal life to tell me what to do and how to run my life."
- "I don't deserve to be loved unconditionally."
- "I can't let others see me sweat. I must look cool."
- "I act stoic, but deep down I am scared."
- "I have to live what my dad wants me to be, not what I want to be."
- "I am insecure."
- "I'm afraid of being hurt."
- "I'm afraid of being trapped in a relationship."
- "Failure is not an option."

CASE STUDY: Ken

Ken's nail biting interfered with the quality of his life in many ways. It was painful, his nails often became infected, and he was embarrassed by how they looked. He was a bank officer, and told me, "I have to keep my hands under the table at meetings. When I have to put them where other people can see them, to write or hand around papers, it's really humiliating."

Ken had opted into this habit as a child, and just didn't seem to be able to stop. Under hypnosis, he realized that his Uncle Fred had routinely made fun of him for his curly hair, and the parents had done nothing to stop Fred. The lesson Ken absorbed was, "I must deserve to be embarrassed and humiliated."

There are lots of ways we can ensure that we are embarrassed and humiliated, but Ken's other, positive self concepts and beliefs facilitated good relationships as well as professional competence. So he did it by turning his nail beds raw at the tips. His stubby, mutilated finger tips humiliated him in front of his peers.

For a time after our initial round of sessions, Ken stopped biting his nails. He was amazed, and very pleased. But six months later, he failed to get a promotion that he expected and took up the habit again. He returned to finish "Cleaning House," and we discovered an ancillary belief: "I deserve to be punished." The way he had punished himself for not getting the promotion was the familiar habit of biting his nails and cuticle. When we dealt with that belief, he was able to stop for good.

EPILOGUE

I began this book by saying that it is about hope. Its purpose is to offer a more advanced and comprehensive way to heal the dis-eases of our times, so as to honor life, live with joy, love wisely and unconditionally, preserve freedom for all, act with compassion and serve the cause of peace.

Core Healing goes beyond simply attempting to fix all that is painful or uncomfortable. It can be the passage into a new life, one where we are free to foster our unique talents and abilities as well as free ourselves to cultivate wholesome relationships and live with a clear sense of Divine embrace.

When each of us engages Core Healing not just to quit smoking, drugging or drinking, not just to cure depression and anxiety problems but more globally for a sense of being at peace within as well as among our neighbors, then, over the next several decades, together, we can heal our world. With such collective commitment, *we become the messiah*. Why not create peace as opposed to Armageddon, as we are now doing through this collective of our subconscious minds (Jung & Campbell, 1976)? Instead, let us live in the truism attributed to Benjamin Franklin, "God helps those who help themselves." Therefore, let us each be responsible for fostering peace within ourselves. That is our only path for an enduring peace with each other.

BIBLIOGRAPHY

These attributions are meant to represent the giants upon whose shoulders Core Healing stands. I humbly salute these my teachers who have influenced the assemblage of Core Healing. Aspects of their work are reflected in the dynamic Core Healing process. Any not listed here, that should be, is a matter of the sin of omission not commission.

Bandler, R., Grinder, J. *Reframing: Neuro-Linguistic Programming and the Transformation of Meaning* (1981); Boulder: Real People Press.

Bandura, Albert. *Social Learning Theory* (1976); New York: Prentice Hall.

Beck, Aaron. T. *Cognitive Therapy and the Emotional Disorders* (1976); Madison, CT: International Universities Press, Inc.

Begley, Sharon. *Train Your Mind, Change Your Brain: How a new science reveals our extraordinary potential to transform ourselves* (2007); New York: Ballantine Books.

Berne, Eric. *Games People Play* (1964); New York: Grove Press.

Brown, Alice J. *Core Beliefs Psychotherapy: Theory and Practice, Second Edition* (2007); Plymouth: Core Healing Center, Inc.

Byrne, Rhonda. *The Secret* (2006); New York: Atria Books; Beyond Words Publishers.

Bradshaw, John. *Homecoming: reclaiming and championing your inner child* (1990); New York: Bantam.

Cheek, David B. *Hypnosis: The application of ideomotor techniques* (1994); Boston: Allyn &Bacon.

Dreikurs, Rudolf. *Happy Children: a challenge to parents* (1972); New York: Fontana Books.

Ellis, Albert. *A New Guide to Rational Living* (1975); New York: Prentice Hall.

Erickson, Milton H. *Life Reframing in Hypnosis* (1985); In E. L. Rossi & M.O. Ryan (Eds.) *The seminars, workshops and lectures of Milton H. Erickson (Vol. 2)*. New York: Irvington.

Ewin,D.M. and Eimer, BN. *Ideomotor Signals for Rapid Hypoanalysis: a how to manual* (2006); Springfield: Charles C. Thomas.

Frances, Allen, M.D., et.al. *Diagnostic and Statistical Manual of Mental Disorders: Fourth edition* (1994); Washington, D.C.: American Psychiatric Association.
Frankl, Victor. *Doctor and the Soul* (1988); Gloucester, MA: Peter Smith Publishers, Inc.
Gardner, J.W. *Excellence* (1961); New York: Harper & Row.
Glasser, William. *Positive Addiction* (1976); New York: Harper Row.
Greenwald, Harold. *Direct Decision Therapy* (1973); San Diego: Edits Publications.
Hammond, Corydon D. *Handbook of Hypnotic Suggestions and Metaphors* (1990); New York: W. W. Norton and Company.
Harris, Judith Rich. *No Two Alike: human nature and human individuality* (2006); New York: W.W. Norton & Co.
Hay, Louise. *Heal Your Body* (1976); Santa Monica: Hay House, Inc.
Jung, C.G., & Campbell, J. *The Portable Jung (a compilation)* (1976); New York: Penguin Books.
Maslow, Abraham. *Toward a Psychology of Being* (1962); New York: Van Nostrand.
Parkhill, Steve. *Answer Cancer* (1995); Deerfield Beach, Florida: Health Communications.
Riese, Hertha. *Heal the Hurt Child* (1966); Chicago: The University of Chicago Press.
Rogers, Carl. *On Becoming a Person: a therapist's view of psychotherapy* (1961); Boston: Houghton Mifflin.
Rossi, Ernest. *The Psychobiology of Mind Body Healing: New concepts in therapeutic hypnosis* (1993); New York: Norton.
Siegel, Bernie. *Love, Medicine and Miracles* (1986); New York: Harper Collins.
Tyrell, Donald J. *Living by Choice* (1977); New York: Philosophical Press, Inc.
Tyrell, Donald J. *When Love Is Lost* (1972); Waco, Texas: Word Books Publisher.
Zarren, Jordan I. and Eimer, Bruce N. *Brief Cognitive Hypnosis: Facilitating the change of dysfunctional behavior* (2002); New York: Springer Publishing Company.